AF207015

TEEN DISORDERS

What Is

ADHD?

By Yvette LaPierre

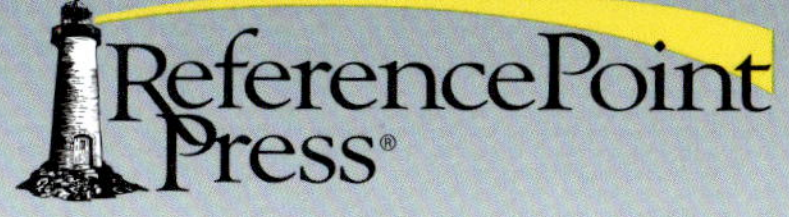

ReferencePoint Press®

San Diego, CA

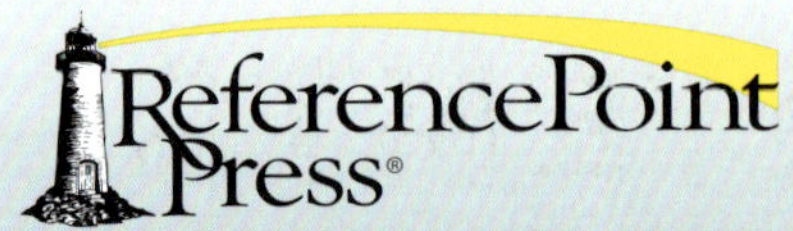

© 2021 ReferencePoint Press, Inc.
Printed in the United States

For more information, contact:
ReferencePoint Press, Inc.
PO Box 27779
San Diego, CA 92198
www.ReferencePointPress.com

ALL RIGHTS RESERVED.

No part of this work covered by the copyright hereon may be reproduced or used in any form or by any means—graphic, electronic, or mechanical, including photocopying, recording, taping, web distribution, or information storage retrieval systems—without the written permission of the publisher.

Content Consultant: Kevin Antshel, Professor, Director of Clinical Training, Psychology, Syracuse University

LIBRARY OF CONGRESS CATALOGING-IN-PUBLICATION DATA

Names: LaPierre, Yvette, 1963- author.
Title: What is ADHD? / by Yvette LaPierre.
Description: San Diego : ReferencePoint Press, [2021] | Series: Teen disorders | Includes bibliographical references and index. | Audience: Grades 10-12
Identifiers: LCCN 2020003557 (print) | LCCN 2020003558 (eBook) | ISBN 9781682829479 (hardcover) | ISBN 9781682829486 (eBook)
Subjects: LCSH: Attention-deficit hyperactivity disorder--Juvenile literature. | Attention-deficit hyperactivity disorder--Diagnosis--Juvenile literature. | Attention-deficit hyperactivity disorder--Treatment--Juvenile literature.
Classification: LCC RJ506.H9 L37 2021 (print) | LCC RJ506.H9 (eBook) | DDC 618.92/8589--dc23
LC record available at https://lccn.loc.gov/2020003557
LC eBook record available at https://lccn.loc.gov/2020003558

CONTENTS

Unable to Focus

"Cara? Cara! Answer the question, please." Cara comes out of the fog of her daydream to find Ms. Johnson and all the students in the class staring at her, and she has no idea what the question is. Cara knows she should pay attention in class, and she tries to. But after a few minutes of listening to the teacher, she finds her mind wandering off to other thoughts. Cara likes learning and works hard on her assignments. But sometimes she loses her homework or forgets the date of a big test. As a result, her grades aren't great. She wants to go to college, but her counselors and teachers keep telling her she'll never get accepted if she doesn't focus and try harder. She begins to think about all the college applications she has started and needs to finish. Suddenly, her teacher's voice snaps her back to the present. "Cara?! Pay attention!"

A WIDESPREAD DISORDER

Many adolescents and teens have trouble sitting still, paying attention, and focusing on tasks at times in their lives. But for people with attention-deficit/hyperactivity disorder (ADHD),

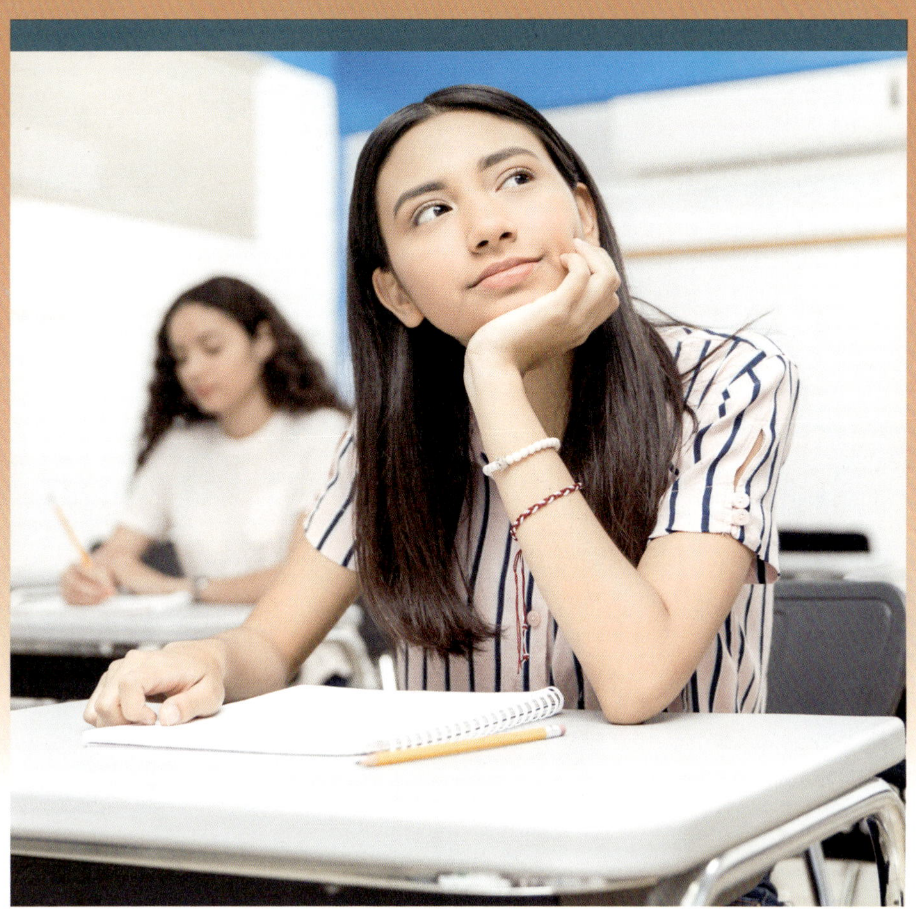

People with ADHD are easily distracted and find it difficult to concentrate. This can make it hard to learn and succeed in school.

these problems are persistent and affect all areas of their lives, from home to school to social activities to friends. According to the Centers for Disease Control and Prevention (CDC), "Millions of US children have been diagnosed with ADHD."[1] It affects at least one in twenty children ages two to seventeen in the United States. That means that in any given classroom, at least one or two students are likely to be dealing with ADHD symptoms. ADHD is a neurodevelopmental disorder. *Neurodevelopmental*

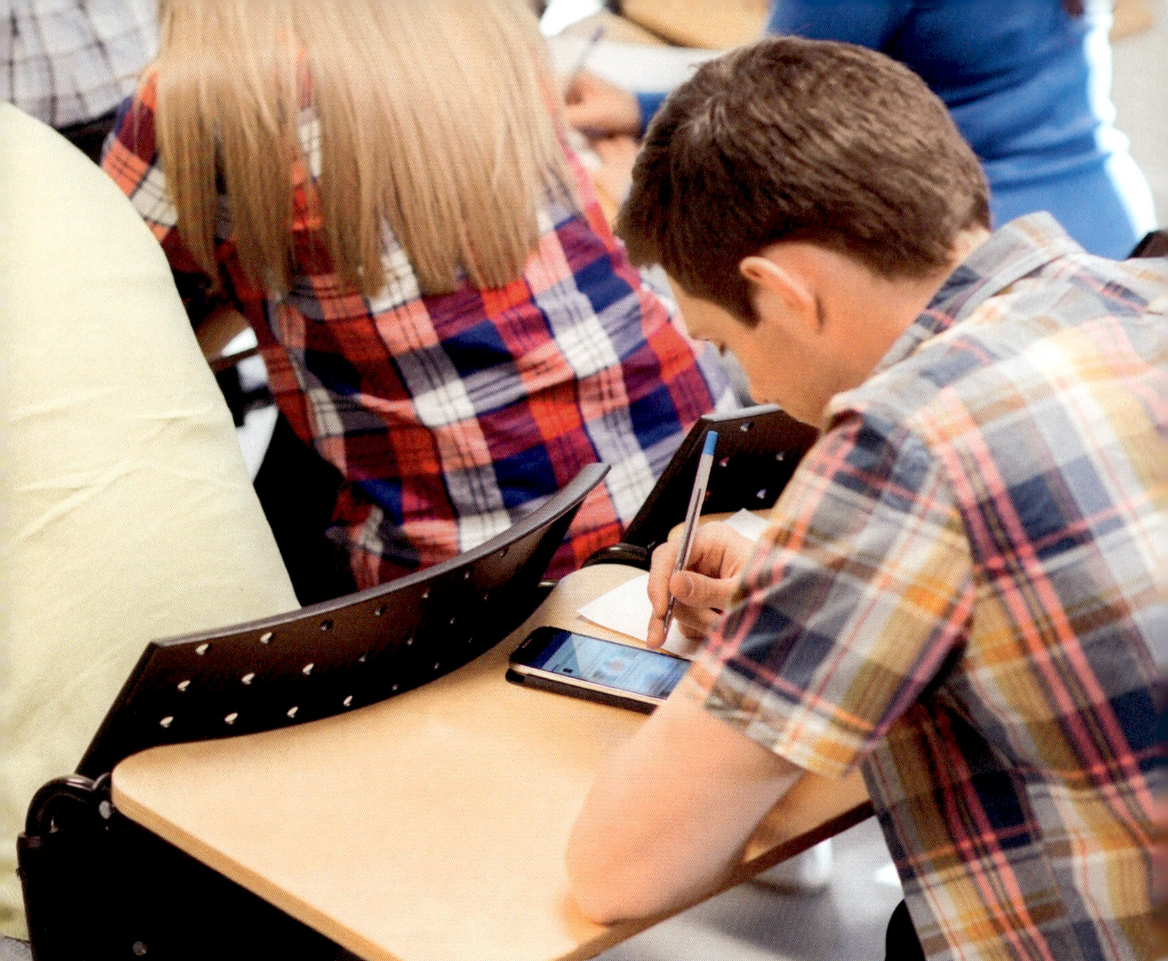

While many people have trouble staying on task, teens with ADHD have an especially difficult time. Attentional problems happen more frequently and are harder to control.

means it is linked to how the brain develops and how it receives, processes, and sends information throughout the body. The brain's development affects many of its functions, including behavior, regulation of emotions, and memory and organization. A delay in neurodevelopment results in the three core symptoms of ADHD: inattention, hyperactivity, and impulsivity. People with ADHD may have one or more of those symptoms.

ADHD is a complex medical condition that requires a specific diagnosis before treatment. Treatment often includes a combination of medication and behavioral therapy. According to the Society of Clinical Child & Adolescent Psychology, "Many of the behavioral problems or mental health symptoms that can keep children and adolescents from leading happy, successful lives can be effectively treated with evidence-based therapies."[2] People with ADHD also can learn coping skills and strategies to manage the symptoms of ADHD. Some children seem to grow out of some of the symptoms of ADHD as they age, but the majority will continue to struggle with these symptoms into adulthood. The teen years can be especially challenging for people with ADHD. Academic and social pressures increase at a time when teens are expected to behave with more responsibility and independence, which can worsen symptoms and heighten frustration levels. With proper diagnosis, treatment, and management, however, many people with ADHD learn to cope and even thrive with the disorder.

> **"Millions of US children have been diagnosed with ADHD."[1]**
> *—CDC*

CHAPTER ONE

What Is ADHD?

The American Psychiatric Association publishes the *Diagnostic and Statistical Manual of Mental Disorders (DSM)*, a publication that helps medical professionals and researchers diagnose and classify mental disorders. The latest edition, known as the *DSM-5*, was published in 2013. In defining ADHD, the *DSM-5* explains, "People with ADHD show a persistent pattern of inattention and/or hyperactivity-impulsivity that interferes with functioning or development."[3]

ADHD is present from birth, but the symptoms often are not noticed by parents or other adults until school age. This may be the first time the child is expected to sit still and pay attention for long periods of time. But some children experience difficulties at home and in social situations before going to school. To diagnose ADHD, several symptoms must be present before age twelve. For some people, ADHD symptoms are never recognized as traits of the disorder. These people may end up never getting diagnosed at all.

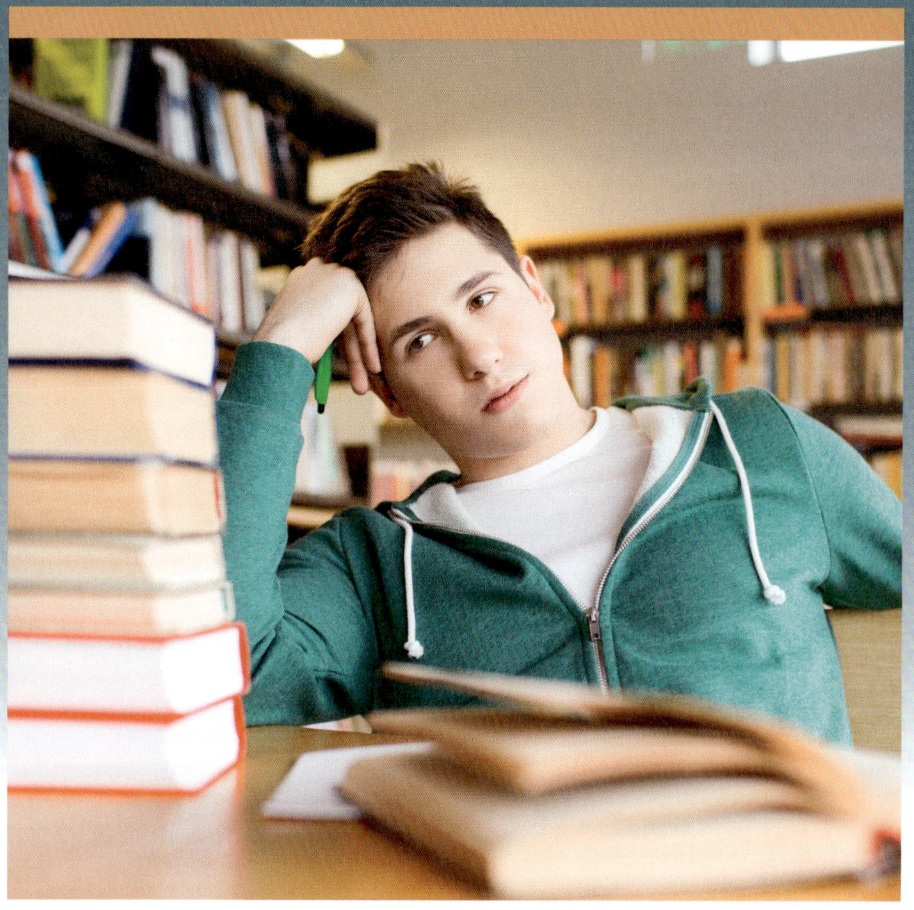

Symptoms of ADHD can range from fidgeting to daydreaming. The symptoms may differ between boys and girls.

ADHD can be difficult to diagnose because many children have trouble sitting still and paying attention, and many children act impulsively at times. This can make it challenging to distinguish between behavior related to a disorder and behavior appropriate to developmental levels. And, of course, every person is unique, so each person will experience symptoms differently. In addition, there are three subtypes of ADHD, so not everyone with the disorder has the same traits. Adolescents with the predominantly hyperactive-impulsive subtype of ADHD tend to be fidgety and active, can't sit still, and talk a lot. Boys are most often diagnosed with this subtype. Those with the predominantly inattentive subtype of ADHD have trouble paying attention and staying focused. Rather than fidgeting in class, they tend to daydream. They also tend to be disorganized and forget things. When girls are diagnosed with ADHD, they tend to be diagnosed with this subtype. The most common type of ADHD for children and teens is the combined type, which is a mix of the traits of hyperactivity, impulsivity, and inattention.

ADD or ADHD?

The correct medical term for the disorder is ADHD, or attention-deficit/hyperactivity disorder. Many people, however, use the term ADD, or attention-deficit disorder. The disorder has been known by many names since it was first described back in the late 1700s. Those names include minimal brain dysfunction, hyperkinetic reaction of childhood, and attention-deficit disorder. As research and understanding of the disorder and its traits have evolved, so has the name. At one time, the condition was called ADD with or without hyperactivity. Now experts label the condition ADHD with three different subtypes. They recognize that people may have one, some, or all of the classic traits of hyperactivity, inattention, and impulsivity.

A BRAIN-BASED DISORDER

ADHD is a neurodevelopmental disorder. This means that it is caused by differences in the growth or development of the

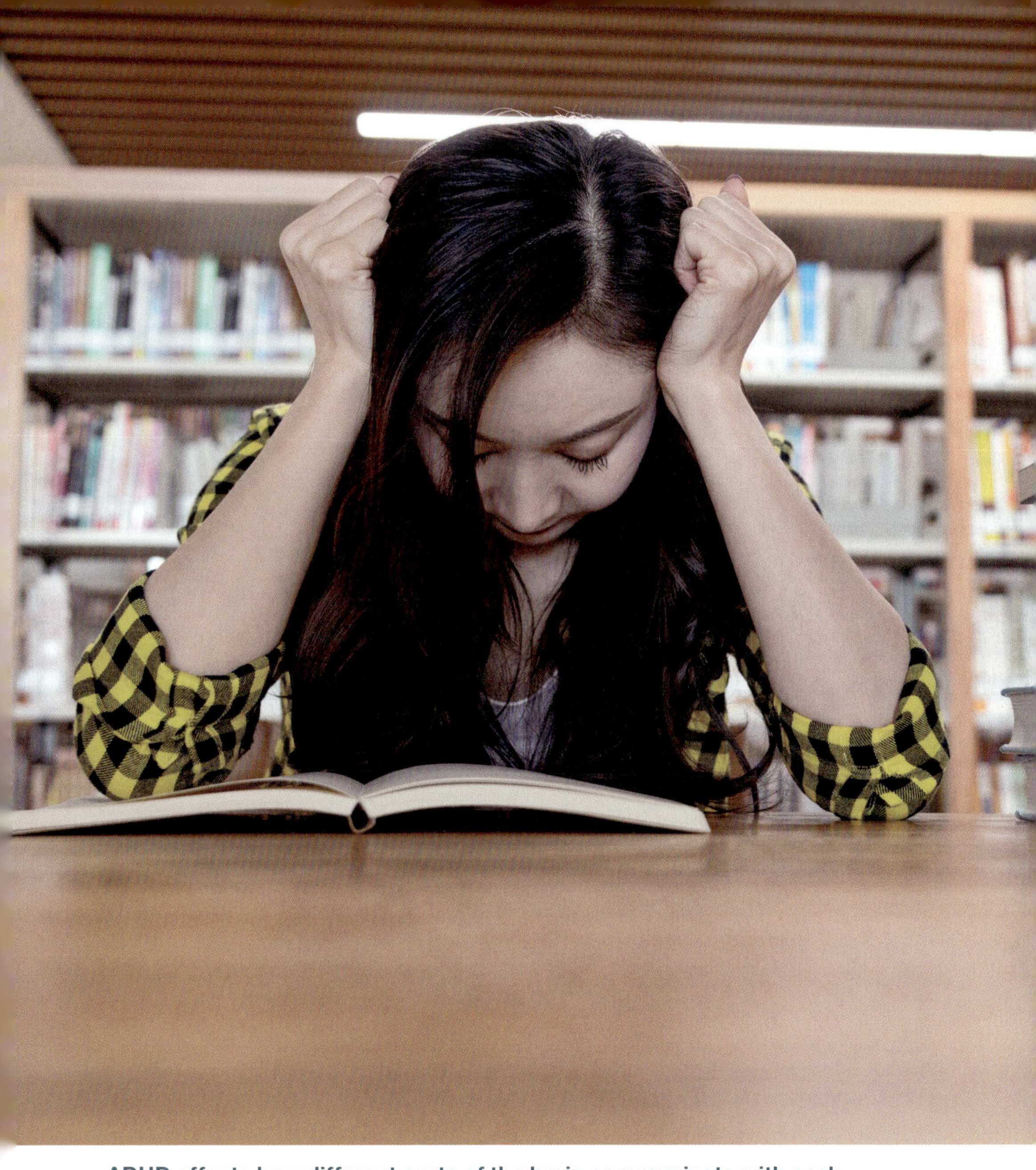

ADHD affects how different parts of the brain communicate with each other. People with ADHD have a lower amount of activity in the parts of the brain that help regulate attention.

brain. Experts believe that the brains of people with ADHD

process information differently than the brains of those without

ADHD. The impaired information processing is what causes

the traits associated with ADHD. Psychologist and author John F. Taylor describes it this way: "It's like a bad telephone connection: Different parts of your brain are trying to 'talk' to one another but the line is full of static and the messages can't get through."[4] ADHD affects areas of the brain that control a set of brain functions known as executive functioning skills. These functions help people engage in goal-directed problem-solving behaviors, and they include attention, concentration, memory, motivation and effort, learning from mistakes, impulse control, organization, and planning, among other important functions.

The brain continues to grow and develop throughout childhood and adolescence. That is why some people seem to grow out of ADHD by young adulthood. The Mayo Clinic notes, "Symptoms sometimes lessen with age. However, some people never completely outgrow their ADHD symptoms."[5] More than three-quarters of children with ADHD continue to experience significant symptoms of ADHD into adulthood. This can cause problems with school, work, and relationships. The cause of the brain development differences appears to be genetic in nature.

Studies show that ADHD tends to run in families. A person with an immediate family member with ADHD, such as a parent or a sibling, is more likely to have ADHD than someone from the general population.

PREVALENCE

According to the CDC, "ADHD is one of the most common neurodevelopmental disorders of childhood."[6] People all over the world have ADHD. Governments and nongovernmental organizations such as the World Health Organization collect data on numbers of people diagnosed with ADHD. In the United States, the CDC and other agencies conduct national surveys to collect statistics on the disorder. Researchers and the health care industry also conduct studies. A number of different studies show that 5 to 10 percent of children in the United States have some form of ADHD. Approximately 2.5 percent of the US adult population has ADHD.

Some studies have concluded that ADHD is more prevalent in males than females. New research, however, suggests that may not be the case. ADHD is diagnosed more often in boys than girls, but it may be that girls are consistently

Kids Will Be Kids?

Throughout history, many people have described the behaviors that characterize ADHD as just kids being kids. After all, many kids are active and impulsive and have trouble sitting still and paying attention. Jonathan Chesner, an actor who wrote a book about his experiences with ADHD, says, "They [cynical people] think ADHD is an excuse and you're just trying to get extended time on your tests or easier grading."[1] Medical researchers have recognized that ADHD is a brain-based disorder since the 1970s, but some people still believe that many cases are simply typical kid behavior that they will grow out of. In 2002, physicians who were concerned about misinformation about ADHD in the media signed an International Consensus Statement on ADHD. The statement asserts, in part: "We cannot overemphasize the point that, as a matter of science, the notion that ADHD does not exist is simply wrong. All of the major medical associations and government health agencies recognize ADHD as a genuine disorder because the scientific evidence indicating it is so overwhelming."[2]

1. Jonathan Chesner, ADHD in HD: Brains Gone Wild. Minneapolis, MN: Free Spirit Publishing, 2012, p. 12.

2. "International Consensus Statement on ADHD." Clinical Child and Family Psychology Review, Vol. 5, No. 2, June 2002, www.russellbarkley.org.

underdiagnosed compared to boys. Boys with ADHD tend to exhibit more hyperactivity, which can lead to behavior issues that are more easily recognized as a problem. Girls with ADHD also have trouble paying attention, but they tend to daydream rather than fidget or cause disruptions in class. As a result, some experts believe that parents and teachers are less likely to recognize that behavior as a symptom of ADHD, meaning many girls with ADHD are not diagnosed.

The CDC conducted the National Health Interview Survey (NHIS) in 2016 and reported the resulting statistics about ADHD in the United States. According to

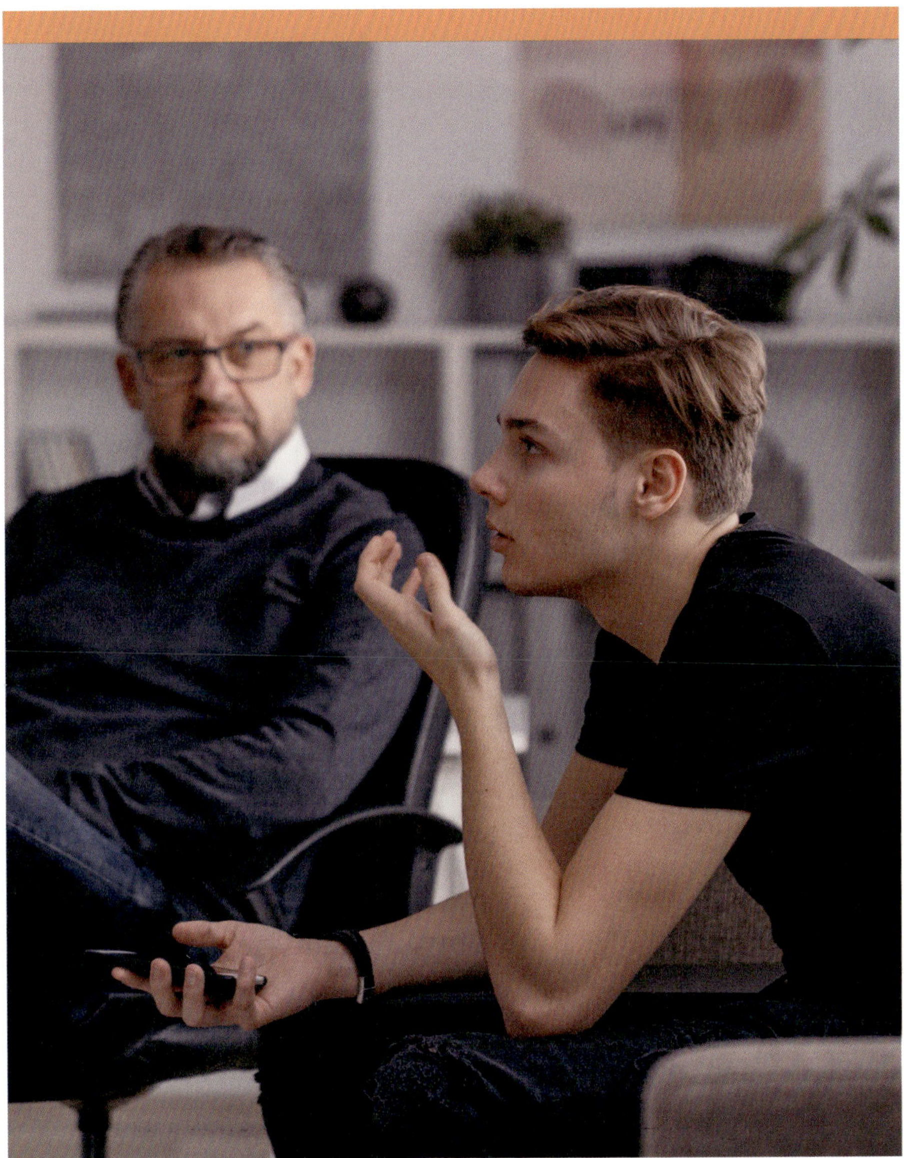

ADHD can be treated with medication and behavioral therapy. Treatment plans help manage symptoms and create lifestyles that benefit mental health.

the survey, 6.1 million children ages two to seventeen living

in the United States had at one point been diagnosed with

ADHD. That is about 10 percent of the entire US population in

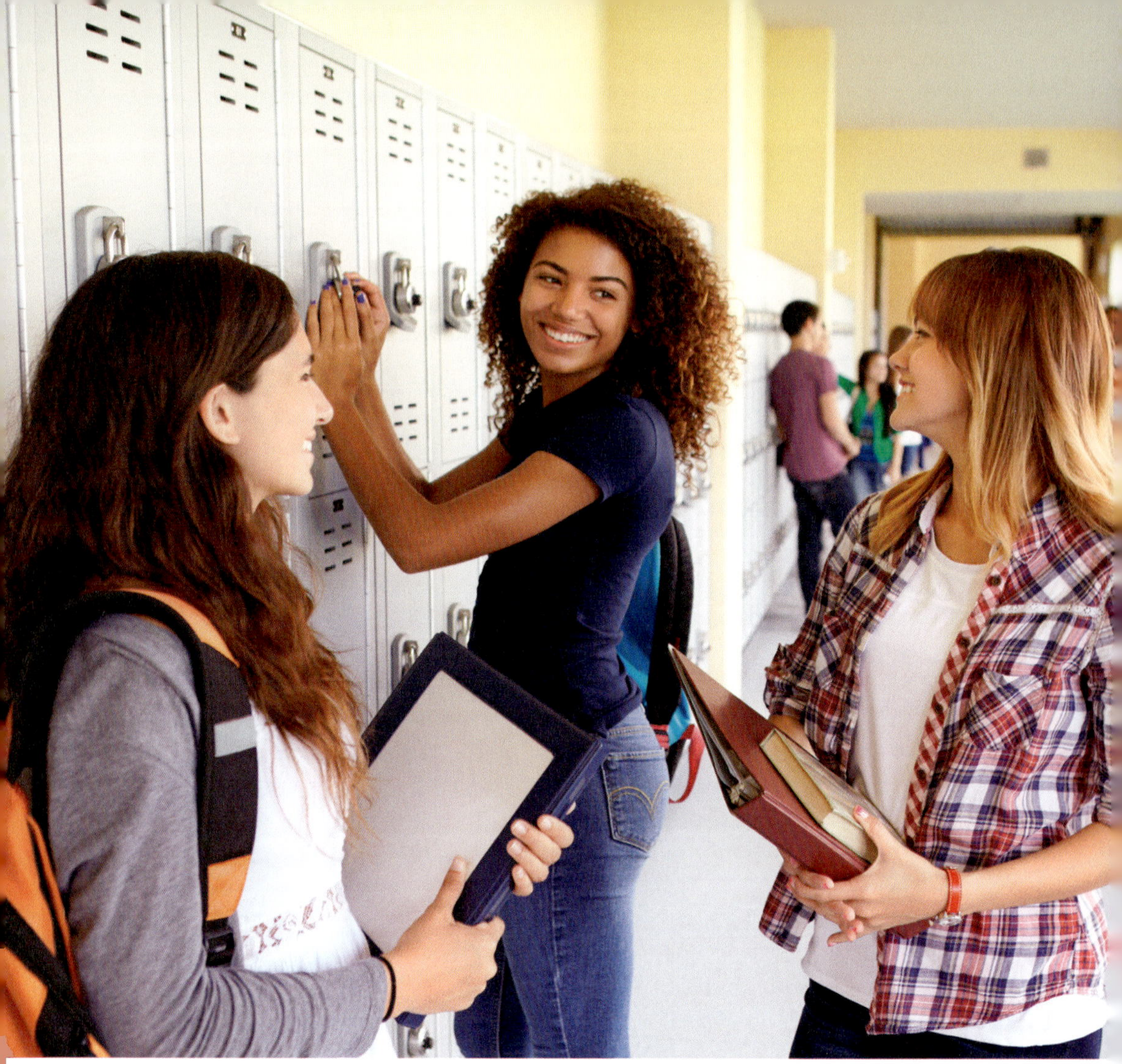

Millions of teens across the United States deal with ADHD. They are treated in a variety of different ways.

that age range. Of those, 388,000 were children ages two to five years, 2.4 million were ages six to eleven years, and 3.3 million were in the twelve to seventeen age range, representing about 13.6 percent of that age group. In 2016, 5.4 million children had a current ADHD diagnosis. That number included 2.9 million kids ages twelve to seventeen, or 11.9 percent of that age group.

The survey also showed that out of the overall number of children with ADHD, 62 percent were taking medication for the disorder. That represents one in twenty children living in the United States. Forty-seven percent received behavioral treatment, and about 32 percent of children received both medication and behavioral treatment. In addition, nearly two-thirds (64 percent) of children with ADHD also had another mental, emotional, or behavioral disorder. Of those, the most prevalent diagnoses were behavior or conduct problems (52 percent) and anxiety (33 percent).

CHAPTER TWO

What Causes ADHD and How Is It Diagnosed?

Scientists have not identified an exact cause for the traits associated with ADHD. There is no single test, such as a blood test or brain scan, that can confirm a diagnosis. However, there are differences in the brains of people with ADHD compared to those who do not have the condition. According to the organization Children and Adults with Attention-Deficit/Hyperactivity Disorder (CHADD), "Research has demonstrated that ADHD has a very strong neurobiological basis."[7] These differences are in the development, volume, and function of key areas of the brain. These differences appear to have a genetic link, but environmental

> "Research has demonstrated that ADHD has a very strong neurobiological basis."[7]
>
> —Children and Adults with Attention-Deficit/Hyperactivity Disorder (CHADD)

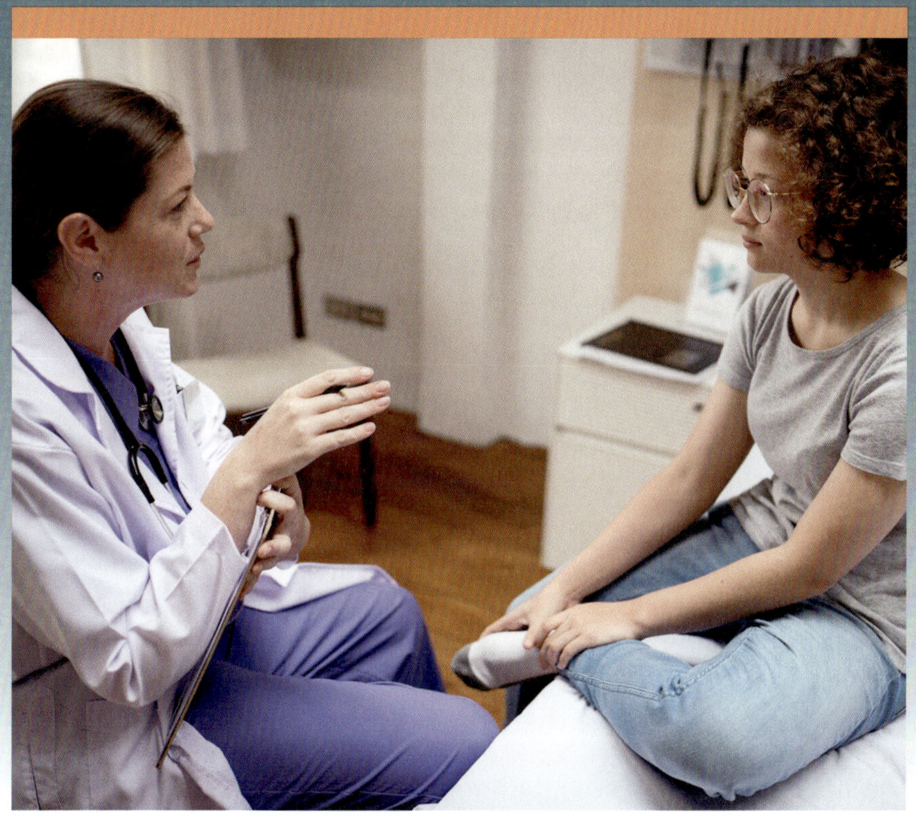

There are many tests that doctors can use to diagnose ADHD. Doctors may ask family members to evaluate their child's behavior or ask the child to take a series of tests that are designed to assess attention.

factors may play a role, too. A thorough understanding of the ADHD brain helps explain the presence of symptoms associated with ADHD and may lead to better diagnostic tools and treatment plans.

THE ADHD BRAIN

New techniques and imaging tools give researchers the ability to look into the brains of people who have ADHD. A large-scale brain imaging study published in 2017 gave scientists the first substantial evidence that people with ADHD have brain structures that differ from those of people without ADHD. The lead researcher of the study commented that she hoped the evidence that ADHD has a basis in the brain, just like other psychiatric disorders, would reach the general public in order to help reduce stigma surrounding the diagnosis.

Scientists have used magnetic resonance imaging (MRI) and other brain imaging technologies to study the development of brains in children with ADHD. A ten-year study by the National Institutes of Health found that brains of children and adolescents with ADHD are 3 to 4 percent smaller than those of children who don't have the disorder. The regions of the brain that are smaller are the areas of the brain that control behavior and cognition. These areas include the frontal, temporal, and parietal lobes, as well as the amygdala. The lobes are associated with different functions ranging from reasoning to interpreting language to sensing touch and pain. The amygdala is the part of the brain responsible for regulating emotions.

In addition to decreased volume in key areas, the ADHD brain connects and communicates differently than the non-ADHD brain. The brain has three main parts: the cerebrum, the cerebellum, and the brain stem. Within those three parts are many more areas that perform various functions. The brain

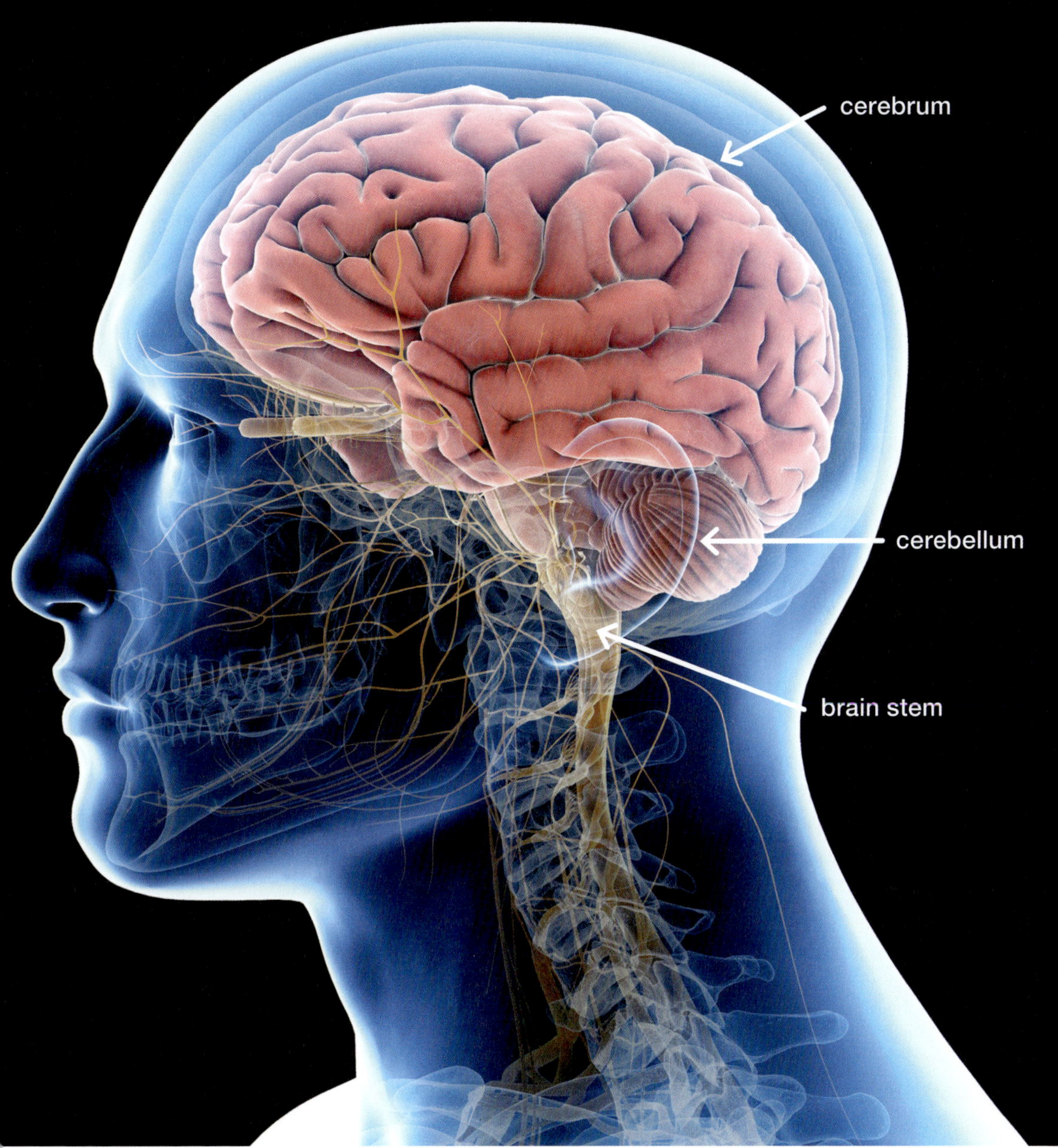

The three main parts of the brain are the cerebrum, the cerebellum, and the brain stem. In people with ADHD, the way these parts connect and communicate is related to the disorder's symptoms.

controls different but completely linked functions. Among these functions are thinking, feeling, perceiving/sensing, physical movement, behaving, and alerting you to danger. For any person

Myths

The traits of ADHD in people have been identified and discussed for hundreds of years. In this time, experts and others have considered many theories about the cause of ADHD. Though researchers don't yet know the exact cause of ADHD, most agree that it is brain linked and highly genetic in nature. And most agree on what does not cause ADHD symptoms. Many earlier theories, however, persist.

For example, one popularly held belief is that ADHD is the result of too much sugar in the diet. But researchers have not found any link between sugar intake and ADHD symptoms. Another common belief is that children develop ADHD as a result of poor parenting. No scientific studies have supported this belief. Researchers also have found no link between family stresses, such as poverty or family conflict, and ADHD traits. Other possible causes of ADHD that are not supported by scientific research include brain injuries, food additives, traumatic life events, and lack of exercise.

Researchers do note, however, that some of these factors might impact the frequency and intensity of ADHD symptoms for some people. For example, too much sugar is not good for anyone's health, and poor general health could aggravate ADHD symptoms. Likewise, exercise can help reduce hyperactivity.

with a brain-based disorder, such as ADHD, at least one of these functions isn't working well. And because all functions within the brain are closely linked, an issue in one area will likely impact other areas.

Each area of the brain communicates with other areas through neurotransmitters. Neurotransmitters are chemicals that carry messages throughout the brain. Studies show that the brains of people with ADHD have low levels of two important neurotransmitters, norepinephrine and dopamine. According to professor of psychiatry Larry Silver, "ADHD was the first disorder found to be

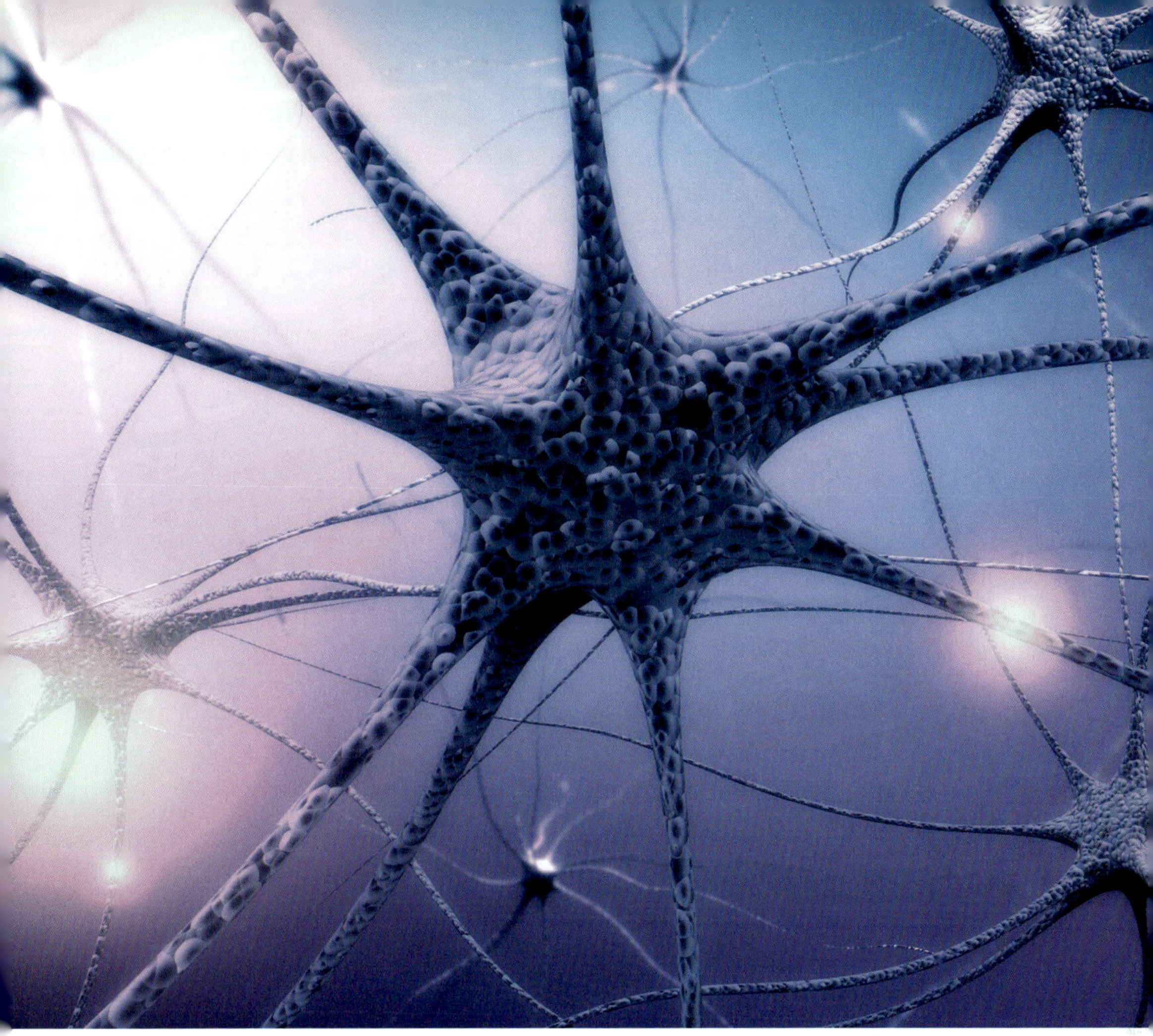

Neurotransmitters help the brain's cells, called neurons (pictured), communicate with one another. A brain has about 100 billion neurons.

the result of a deficiency of a specific neurotransmitter—in this case, norepinephrine."[8] As a result, people with ADHD process information differently than those without it.

This faulty processing and other structural differences impair activity in four important regions of the ADHD brain. The first is the frontal cortex. This region of the brain controls executive functions. The second area impacted is the limbic system, which regulates emotions and attention. Another affected area is the basal ganglia. Reduced activity here can impair information processing and communication within the brain. The last area impacted is the reticular activating system, which is a major system for relaying messages along pathways in the brain.

BRAIN DEVELOPMENT

Much is now known about ADHD brains, but scientists don't yet know why these brains develop differently. The exact cause or causes may be genetic, environmental, or a combination of the two. Many studies show that ADHD tends to run in families, which points to a strong genetic link. Studies suggest that 40 to 60 percent of children who have a parent with ADHD will also have the condition. Several genes have been linked to ADHD, and scientists are working to confirm those findings. Genes are like a set of blueprints, or instructions, that are inherited from biological parents. They are found in every cell of the body. Genes help determine thousands of individual traits, including how a person looks and acts. If researchers can identify specific genes that make people more likely to develop ADHD symptoms, they can focus on better management and preventive treatments.

Some studies throughout the years also have indicated a relationship between ADHD and various environmental

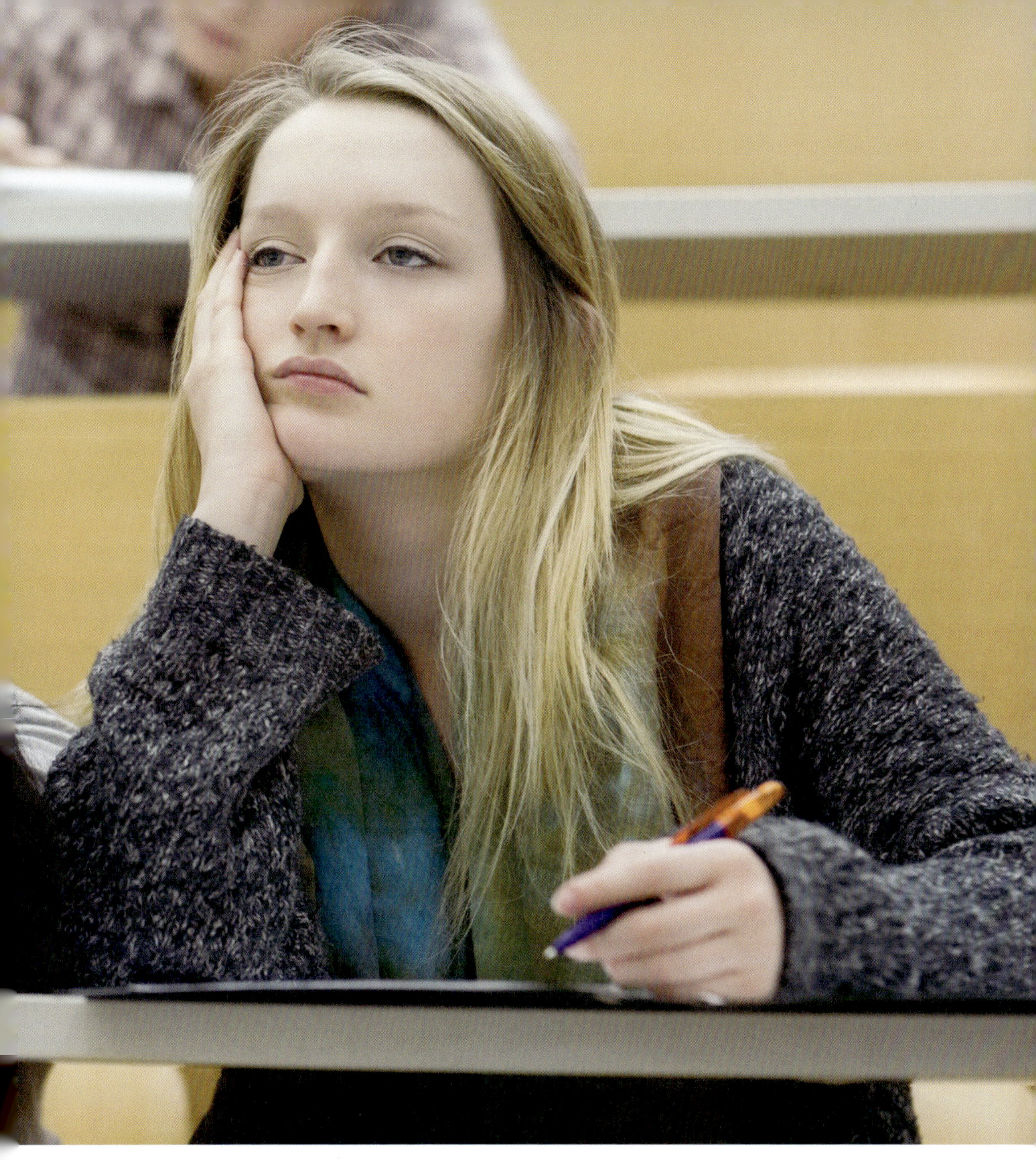

factors. These factors include alcohol and tobacco use during pregnancy, exposure to lead or pesticides during early childhood, and premature birth or low birth weight.

Scientists continue to study the exact causes of ADHD and note that there is likely no single cause for all cases of ADHD.

Scientists have clear evidence that the brains of people with ADHD differ from other brains in both structure and function. The studies don't prove that these anatomical differences cause ADHD. But they do show that the disorder is real and that the ADHD brain behaves differently, resulting in ADHD symptoms.

SYMPTOMS

It's normal for people, especially children and adolescents, to feel distracted at times or so excited that they can't sit still. For most people, though, the feeling or situation ends, and they can get back to a comfortable level of attention and focus. For people with ADHD, however, feeling distracted or hyperactive isn't always tied to a specific event. People with ADHD may feel this way much of the time and in all kinds of situations, including at home and school, during activities, and while hanging out with friends. The ADHD brain can make it hard to focus, remember things, think before acting, stop talking, and follow directions. People with ADHD want to pay attention, but their brains make it hard to do so.

There is no typical child or teen with ADHD. Everyone with ADHD has different symptoms and experiences them differently, according to their individual case. In addition, symptoms can

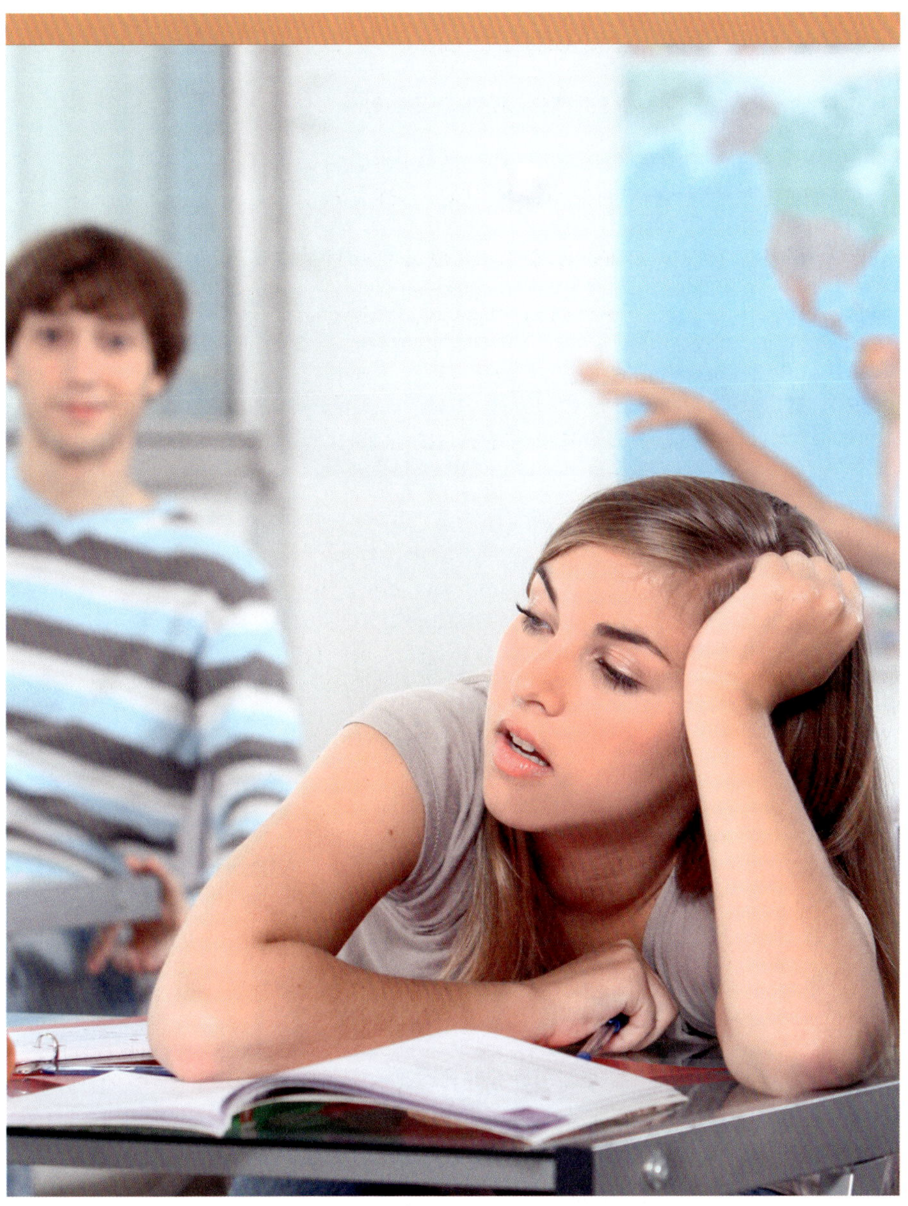

Boredom and misbehavior are not uncommon behaviors in adolescents. They can also be symptoms of ADHD.

vary according to many other factors, such as their gender, the environment they are in, and any other disorders or health issues they may have. Many symptoms mimic some typical behaviors seen in children and adolescents, such as fidgeting and getting bored easily. This can make it difficult for people with ADHD and those around them to separate ADHD symptoms from other developmentally appropriate behaviors. Jonathan Chesner, an actor, entrepreneur, and author who was diagnosed with ADHD at age nine, describes his brain this way: "One way to describe it was that I had the type of brain that would wear a Hawaiian shirt, bright red pants, and cool painted shoes to a wedding."[9]

According to experts, many of the symptoms associated with ADHD are actually symptoms of problems with executive function in the brain. Clinical psychologist Thomas E. Brown of the University of Southern California compares ADHD symptoms resulting from executive function impairments to an orchestra without a conductor. He writes, "Imagine a symphony orchestra in which each musician plays his or her instrument very well. If there is no conductor to organize the orchestra . . . the orchestra will not produce good music."[10] When the brain is not able to coordinate all its functions well, it results in three main symptoms that characterize ADHD, as classified by the *DSM-5*. People with ADHD may exhibit one or more of these symptoms.

The first core symptom is inattention. People who struggle with inattention have trouble staying focused and are easily distracted. As a result, they have trouble finishing projects, following directions, and organizing their day. They may forget and lose important things. An inattentive teen will struggle to finish homework assignments and chores and may forget about important tests or forget to turn in homework. They may daydream during class. Other people may accuse those with ADHD of refusing to listen, follow directions, or remember things. They may say they are lazy, impatient, or have a short attention span.

The next symptom is hyperactivity. The main symptom of hyperactivity is an inability to sit still when asked. People with ADHD may move constantly. They may squirm or tap their fingers or feet while sitting or get up, walk around, and touch things. They may talk excessively or make sounds with their mouths. Teens with ADHD report feeling constantly restless. Hyperactivity makes it difficult to enjoy relaxing or quiet activities or to sit still and quietly in class. Others may call people with these symptoms "hyper" or "fidgety."

The third symptom is impulsivity. People with this trait may speak or act without first thinking about the consequences. They may blurt out inappropriate comments or interrupt when others are talking. They may have trouble waiting their turn. Some may appear overly emotional. All of these symptoms can make relationships with friends and family challenging. Teens with impulsivity may make decisions too quickly without thinking through the best plan. To others, a teen with impulsivity may appear careless or rude.

The presence of some of the symptoms that are associated with ADHD does not mean that an individual has ADHD. Typical adolescent and teen behavior often can be confused with ADHD. Other conditions also can be confused with ADHD, such as learning disabilities, vision or hearing problems, depression, and stress. Physical conditions such a thyroid disorder also can result in ADHD-like symptoms. In addition, ADHD is a very complex disorder that affects individuals in many different ways, and there is no simple test that can confirm a diagnosis. All this makes the diagnosis of ADHD a very complicated process that requires the help of a medical doctor or other trained health provider.

ASSESSMENT PROCESS

Often, the first step is that parents, teachers, or the individual may sense that something is different. As Jonathan Chesner writes in his book *ADHD in HD*, "I was really young when I realized my brain wasn't like other people's brains."[11] A primary care doctor may identify some signs of ADHD and make the diagnosis himself or herself. Or, the doctor may refer the patient to a mental health professional or other doctor who is trained to

accurately assess and diagnose ADHD. A diagnosis requires an extensive interview with the person experiencing the symptoms. In addition, it is important to gather information from others in the patient's life, such as parents and teachers. A comprehensive medical examination is needed to rule out other health issues. In addition, trained health care providers use standardized screening tools to measure ADHD symptoms. For example, continuous performance tests (CPTs) are neuropsychological assessments that measure attention and inhibition. The person being assessed may be asked to perform a task on a computer as a way to measure impulse control, attention, and focus.

Many scales designed to rate symptoms of ADHD are filled out by parents and teachers. These scales take five to fifteen minutes to complete and require the individual to remember how often certain behaviors occur. As a result, while usually reliable, these scales are not always objective and may lead to errors. For example, if a teacher thinks a student is too hyper in class and would benefit from medication, he or she may

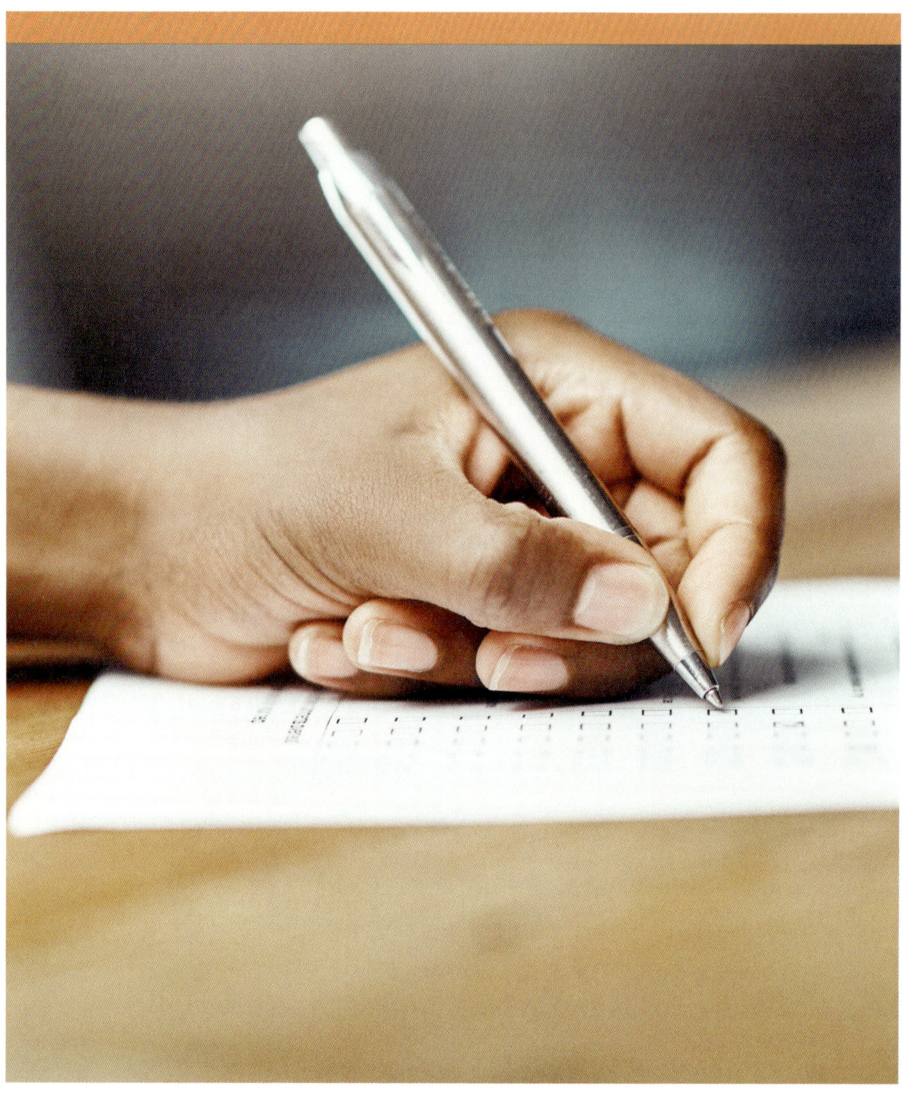

Teachers and parents may be asked to fill out a scale to determine the severity of ADHD symptoms. However, these tests can be biased.

score the symptom as "a severe problem" that occurs "all the time." If parents are reluctant to have their child diagnosed or medicated, they may be tempted to rate symptoms as rarely or never present.

Many experts are looking for more objective methods to measure ADHD symptoms. One example is a quantitative test that measures brain wave patterns to assess attention levels while the patient is performing a task. Another example is the use of a computer that analyzes head movements and facial expressions as the patient completes a task that requires attention. Technology companies have developed virtual reality tools that are a type of CPT. The child puts on a headset and is transported to a virtual classroom. In this virtual classroom, the child sits at a desk, cars drive by outside, paper airplanes glide by,

Social Media and ADHD

A 2018 study published in the *Journal of the American Medical Association* found a link between excessive screen time and the development of symptoms of ADHD in teens. Researchers asked tenth-grade students in California about their digital media use and their self-reported symptoms that could indicate ADHD. The symptoms students were asked about included traits such as difficulty completing tasks and trouble sitting still. The study found a positive link between media use and the development of ADHD symptoms.

The researchers note, however, that the study does not prove that screen time causes ADHD. It could be that students who already show ADHD traits tend to check their phones more frequently. Still, the researchers say that the results should not be ignored. The researchers warn that the constant "pinging" of text messages and other notifications "could disrupt normative development of sustained attention and organization skills." In addition, the ability to access information at any time online "could disrupt development of impulse control and patience."

Jamie Ducharme, "Teens Who Are Constantly on Their Phones May Be at Risk of ADHD, Study Says," Time, July 2018, time.com.

and classmates sneeze. Children being tested are asked to hit a button when certain letters appear on a virtual chalkboard. A computer measures accuracy and reaction speed and how often the child looks at distractions.

DIAGNOSIS

The *DSM-5* defines ADHD and outlines the diagnosis of the disorder in an effort to make the diagnosis more reliable. The *DSM-5* recognizes that symptoms may change over a person's lifetime. For example, symptoms of hyperactivity and impulsivity often lessen as a child with ADHD grows older.

The *DSM-5* lists eighteen core symptoms under two main categories, or domains, of ADHD. Symptoms listed under inattention include often making careless mistakes in schoolwork, often not seeming to listen when spoken to, and often being forgetful. Symptoms under hyperactivity and impulsivity include often fidgeting or squirming in one's seat, talking excessively, and interrupting or intruding on others. For a definite diagnosis, a child must have the onset of six or more symptoms in at least one of these two categories before the age of twelve. In addition, these symptoms must have persisted for at least six months and negatively impacted the child's life in two or more settings. These settings include school,

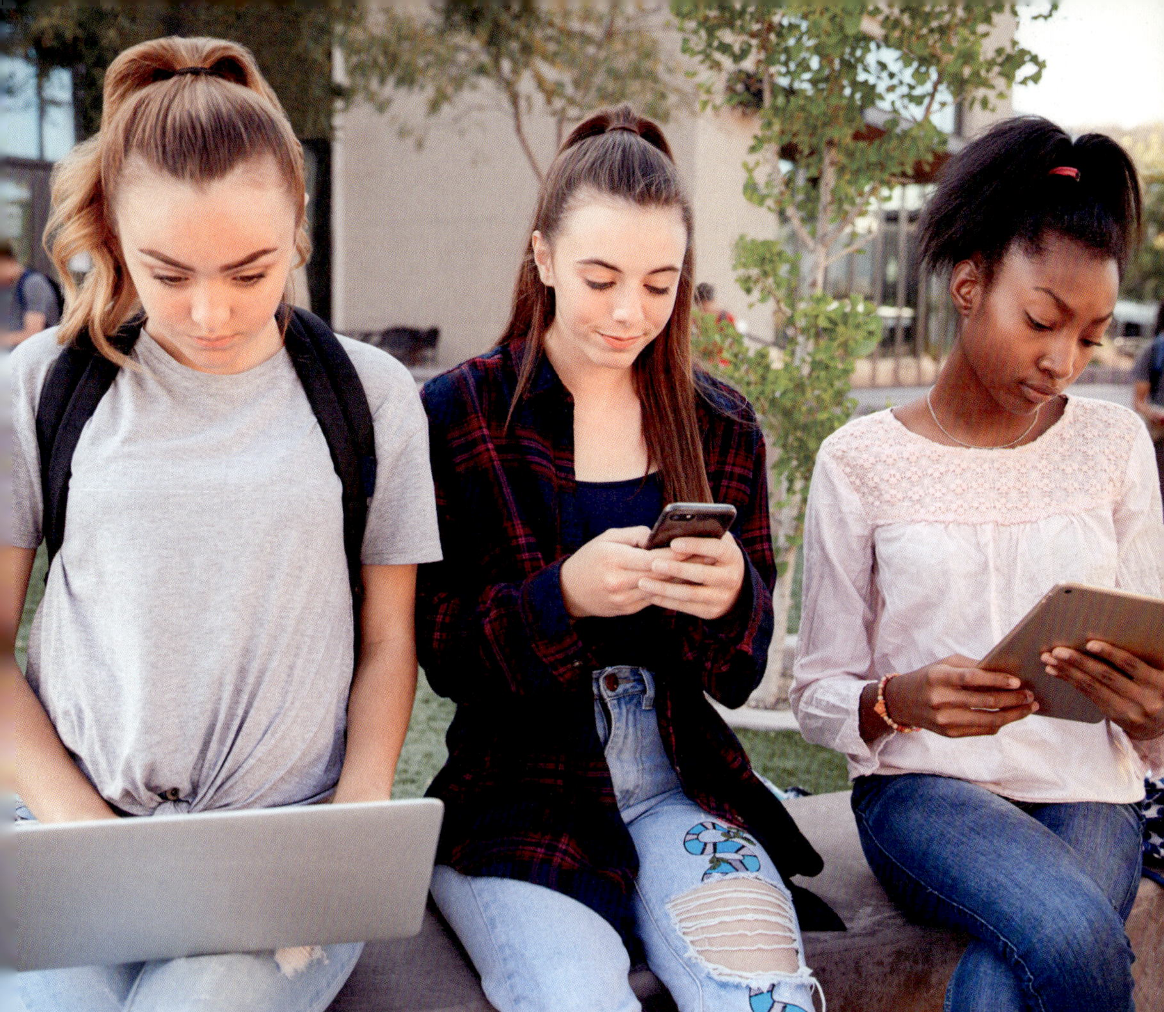

Researchers are studying links between ADHD and social media. More work still needs to be done in this area.

home, and social settings. Teens and adults must have at least five of the symptoms.

Based on the types of symptoms present, the *DSM-5* requires that medical professionals diagnose people with one of three types of ADHD: Predominantly Inattentive, Predominantly Hyperactive/Impulsive, or Combined Presentation (both

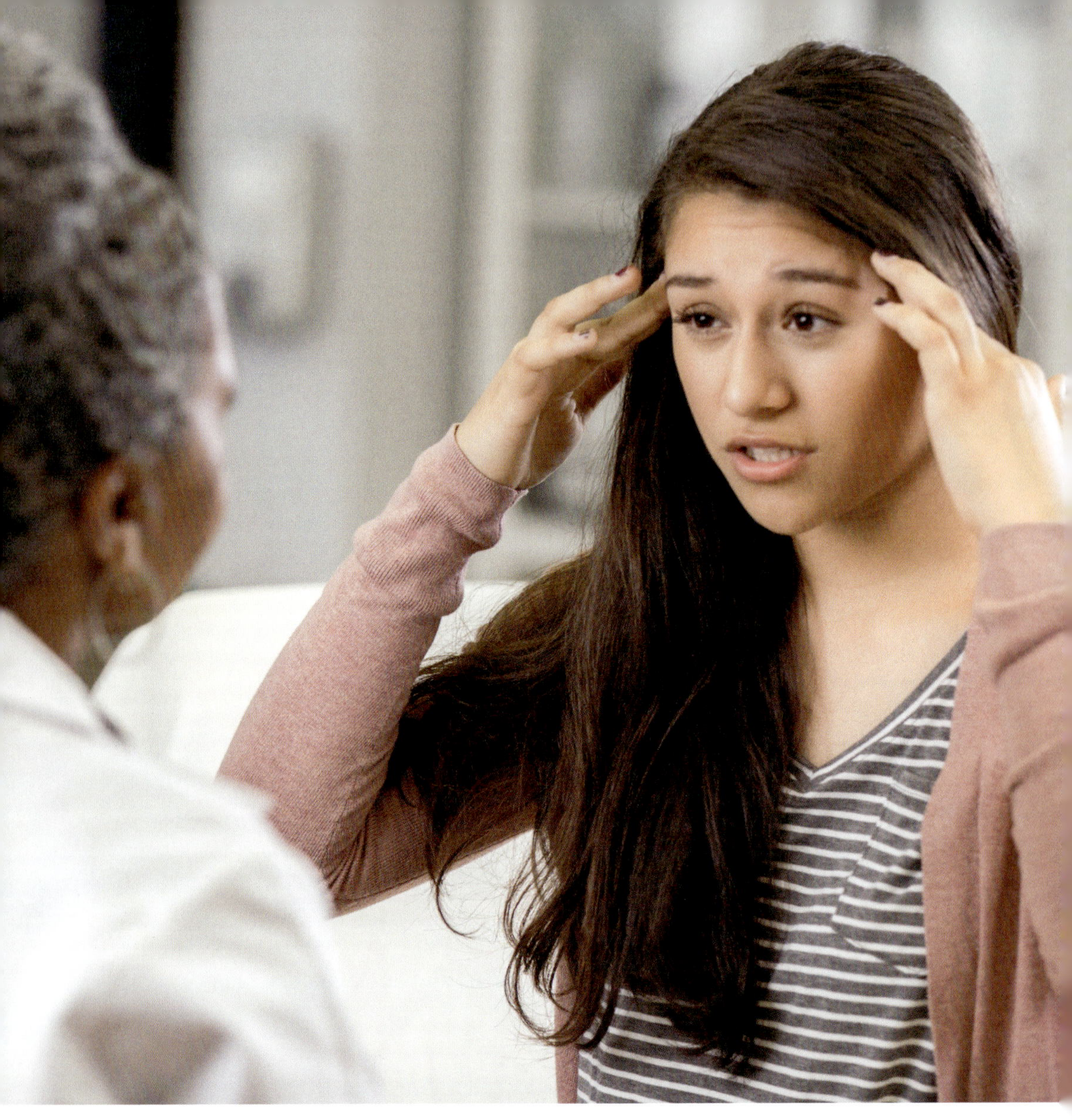

An ADHD diagnosis can help someone identify the cause of their attentional difficulties. The diagnosis is also helpful in identifying treatment plans.

inattentive and hyperactive). Clinicians must also diagnose the person's disorder as mild, moderate, or severe.

A diagnosis of ADHD can be devastating for some people and their loved ones. For others, it can be a relief. A diagnosis is proof that a child or teen is not willfully misbehaving but is dealing with a disorder that can make staying focused and attentive and controlling emotions and impulses difficult, which impacts daily life. It also is important to note that some of the characteristics of ADHD can be positive, too. That's why Jonathan Chesner calls the brains of people with ADHD "special."[12]

CHAPTER THREE

What Is It like to Live with ADHD?

Living with ADHD presents difficulties for people of all ages. The teen years, however, can present a particular challenge. Teens diagnosed with ADHD tend to experience fewer of the hyperactivity symptoms than children with the diagnosis do. But the teen years come with increased academic and life demands, along with many developmental issues, such as establishing independence and dealing with peer pressure. These issues can be particularly tough for teens with ADHD. According to CHADD, "Children with ADHD are at risk for potentially serious problems in adolescence and adulthood: academic failure or delays, driving

> "Children with ADHD are at risk for potentially serious problems in adolescence and adulthood: academic failure or delays, driving problems, difficulties with peers and social situations, risky sexual behavior, and substance abuse."[13]
>
> —CHADD

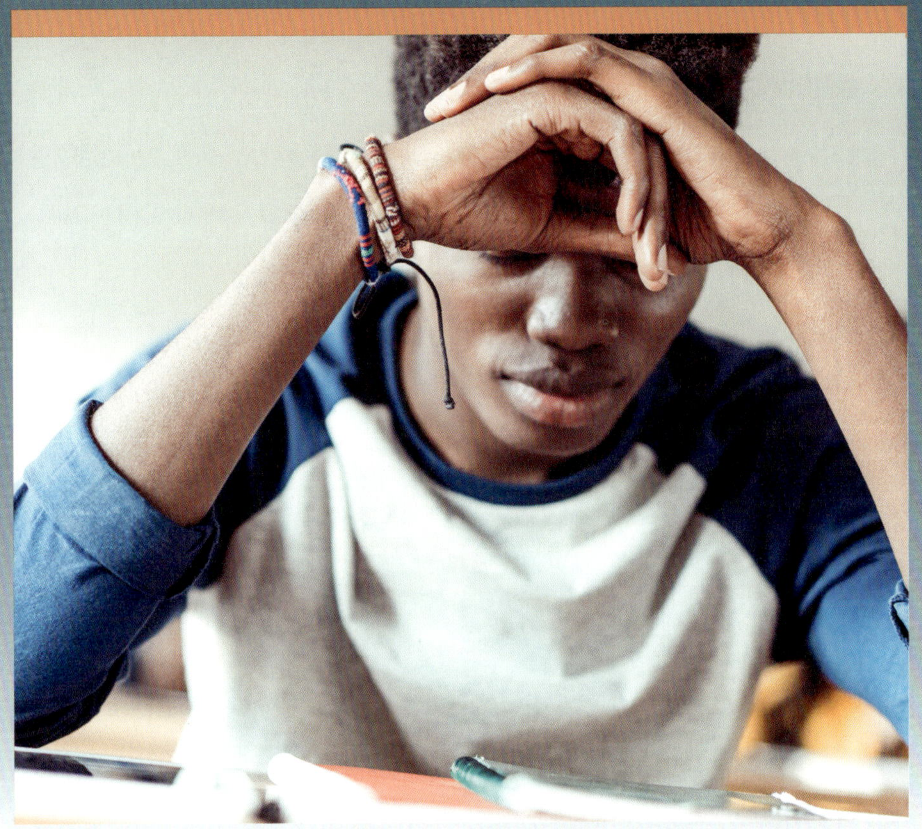

People with ADHD struggle with their disorder throughout their lives. They may have difficulties in school or have social and emotional challenges.

problems, difficulties with peers and social situations, risky sexual behavior, and substance abuse."[13]

MENTAL HEALTH AND TEENS

Many people experience some mental health issues during the teen years. Dr. Stan Kutcher, an expert in adolescent mental health, writes, "Having good mental health makes it easier for you to cope with stress and live your life the way you want to."[14] Changing hormone levels and pressures from school and friends can lead to emotional highs and lows. One associated feature of

Smartphone Addiction

A study of South Korean high school and middle school students with ADHD found that they are at least six times more likely to develop a smartphone addiction than their peers without ADHD, likely due to their impaired impulse control. The authors studied the association between smartphone addiction and symptoms of depression, anxiety, and ADHD, and they reported that the presence of ADHD demonstrated the strongest association with smartphone addiction. They also found that the rate of smartphone addiction was higher in females compared to males.

The authors of the study note that excessive smartphone use has been associated with numerous psychiatric problems, including depression and anxiety. They further note that people ages fourteen to twenty are at particular risk from these negative effects because studies show they are on their cell phones the most. The authors say that "it is particularly important that the effect of smartphone addiction during adolescence should be investigated to implement effective prevention and management plans."

Seung-Gon Kim et al, "The Relationship Between Smartphone Addiction and Symptoms of Depression, Anxiety and Attention-Deficit/Hyperactivity in South Korean Adolescents," Annals of General Psychiatry, December 2019, https://annals-general-psychiatry. biomedcentral.com.

ADHD is difficulty regulating emotions. As a result, teens with ADHD can experience even greater emotional highs and lows than their peers without ADHD, which can make it difficult for them to deal with these issues and can be tough on those around them. For many teens with ADHD, mental health issues develop. Research shows that adolescents and teens with ADHD are at an elevated risk for developing mood disorders, such as anxiety, depression, and bipolar disorder. One study found adolescent girls with ADHD have a 2.5 times higher risk of major depression than those without ADHD.

While teens are dealing with an emotional roller coaster and possible mental health issues, they are expected to handle more responsibility and independence than when they were younger. High school brings higher academic and social demands. At the same time, there is less oversight by teachers and parents to make sure that students are finishing assignments, keeping up with coursework, and staying organized. As teens begin to separate from their parents and other adults in positions of authority, they may become more susceptible to peer pressure, both good and bad. For teens with ADHD, the increase in responsibilities and independence can lead to struggles in daily life.

DEALING WITH STIGMA

Most people want to feel like they fit in and to be liked by their peers and others. Unfortunately, people with ADHD live with both the challenges of ADHD and the stigma associated with it. Kutcher explains, "Stigma is a 'polite' word for discrimination. It's a negative attitude people have about something they don't understand that can result in physical, mental, and emotional harm."[15]

"Stigma is a 'polite' word for discrimination. It's a negative attitude people have about something they don't understand that can result in physical, mental, and emotional harm."[15]

—Dr. Stan Kutcher, expert in adolescent mental health

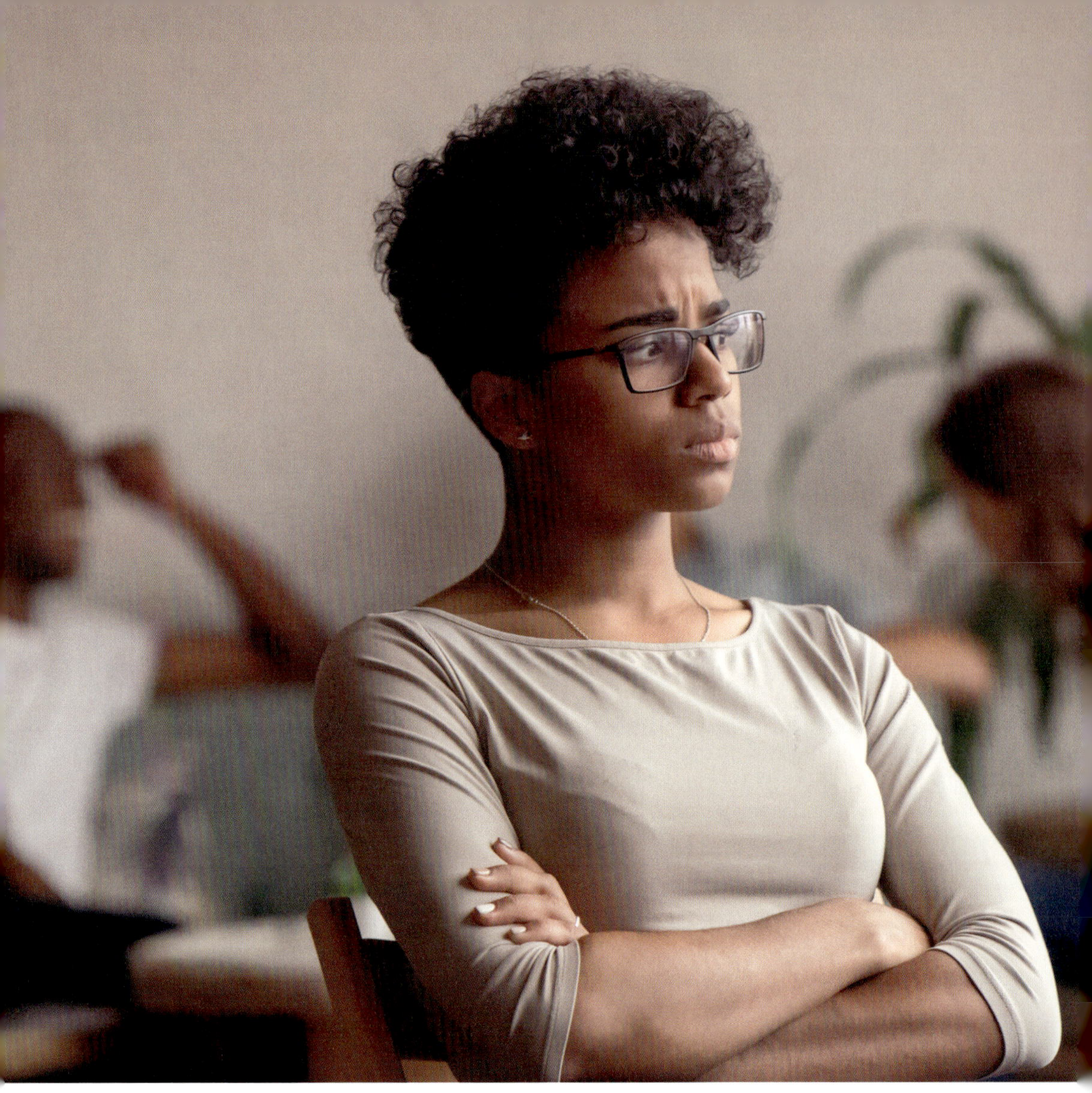

Teenagers with ADHD may be seen as lazy or unintelligent by their classmates. This can be very damaging to their self-esteem and motivation.

People with ADHD may overhear insensitive remarks or feel misunderstood and harshly judged by others. It can be very frustrating and upsetting for someone with ADHD to have their traits constantly mistaken for "bad" behavior. Stuart Passmore, author of *The ADHD Handbook*, describes a study of people with ADHD who report being told repeatedly that they were "problem children": "More specifically, they were told that they were stupid, lazy, and disruptive."[16] Others may say insensitive things because they don't understand ADHD or recognize it as a medical condition. Experts counsel people with ADHD to try not to take such comments personally, but that, of course, is easier said than done.

ACADEMICS

The need for focus, organization, and attention to detail increases as students move from elementary school to middle school to high school and beyond. High school assignments and material are often complex, and students must be able to focus for long periods of time and to follow directions. In-class and nightly assignments often are replaced with long-term assignments that require planning and organization skills. In addition, students must plan ahead, remain focused, and remember large amounts of information for midterms and finals, college entrance exams, and other types of standardized testing. Yet these are the types of skills that many people with ADHD struggle with due to the way their brains function.

Issues with inattention and organization can lead to many problems in school. High school students with ADHD may fail to follow directions carefully or pay attention to details, resulting

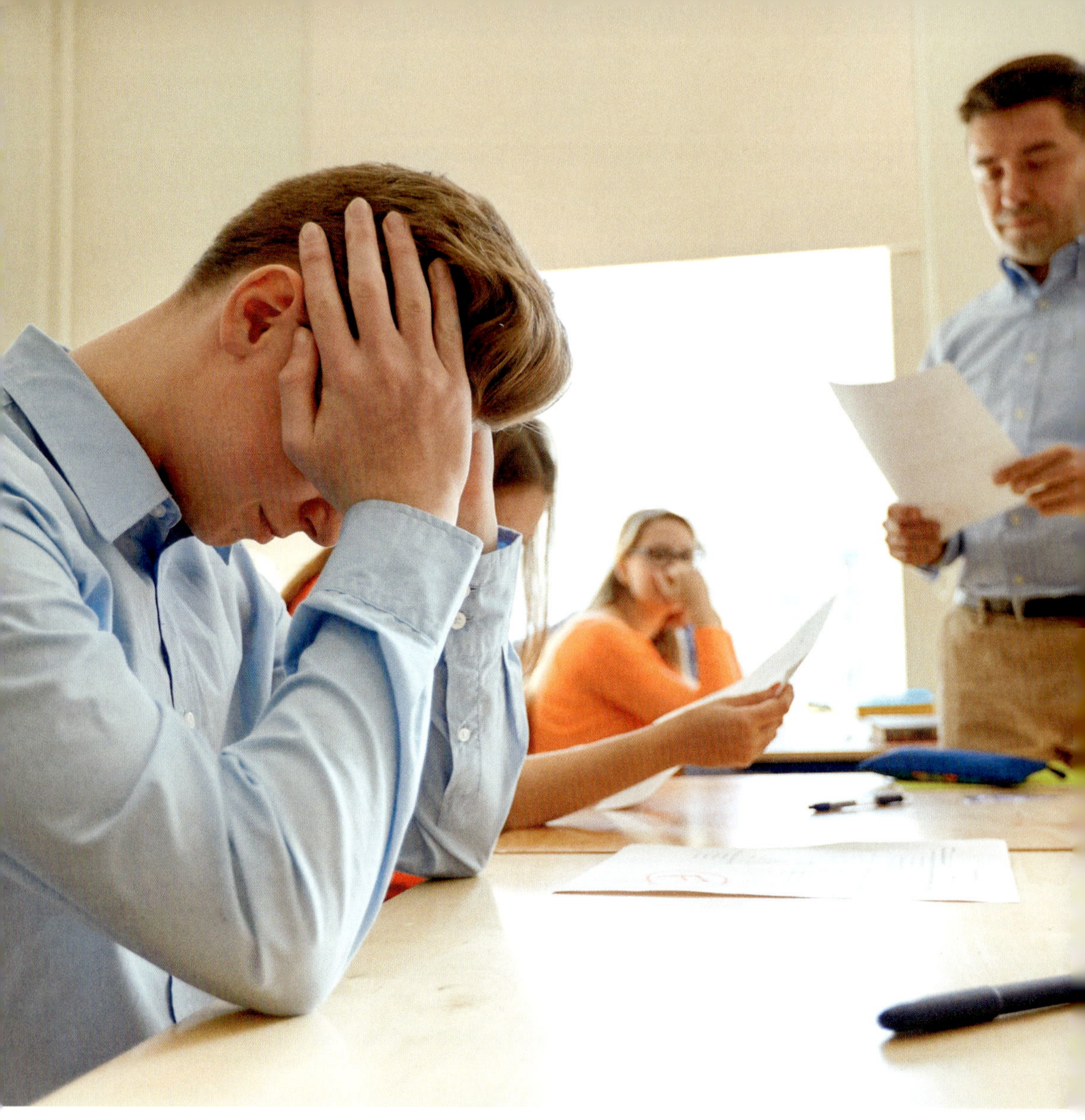

Teachers can make changes in their classrooms to help students with ADHD. They may provide written as well as verbal instruction, break assignments into smaller parts, or provide hands-on activities.

in what might seem like careless mistakes. Inattentiveness may cause students to miss important information or instructions, procrastinate starting a difficult assignment, or jump from task to task without completing one. Impaired organization may result in students forgetting to turn in homework or missing important due dates or tests. Teachers and peers may become frustrated with these students because they appear lazy, unmotivated, or uninterested in school.

Studies show that, without support, teens with ADHD tend to have lower GPAs and standardized test scores than other students, as well as poorer reading skills. As a result, they repeat grades at a higher rate. ADHD also is associated with higher rates of suspension and expulsion for behavioral and academic problems. People with ADHD have lower high school graduation rates, which can lead to reduced employment opportunities throughout their lives.

Students who have been diagnosed with ADHD can take advantage of resources that their schools and communities offer to help them with organization, self-discipline, and general studying and test-taking skills. Tutors and other trained professionals can help with specific class material and academic issues, such as note taking, critical reading, and test anxiety. According to Kutcher, "For someone with ADHD, having a good support system of trusted people is essential."[17]

"For someone with ADHD, having a good support system of trusted people is essential."[17]

—Dr. Stan Kutcher, expert in adolescent mental health

In addition, students with ADHD can request accommodations in school and testing, if needed. Accommodations may include extended time to complete an assessment or test, a quiet place to study or take a test without distractions, or a seat at the front of the classroom. Some students with ADHD are reluctant to request accommodations because it may lead to stigma. As Chesner writes, "One thing that is sort of a drag about extended time is having to take the test by yourself in the library or in a special place for extended-time students. It can feel pretty ostracizing and uncomfortable."[18]

RELATIONSHIPS

All people—from children to adults—sometimes have trouble getting along with friends and family. Research shows, however, that as many as 50 percent of adolescents with ADHD

Driving with ADHD

Studies have found that driving can be a risky activity for teens with ADHD. Teens with ADHD get into accidents and receive traffic tickets more than their peers without ADHD. They are more likely to speed, not wear a seatbelt, and drive while intoxicated. A 2016 study suggests that teens with ADHD get into more accidents while driving because of their hyperactivity, impulsivity, and inattention. They may be more easily distracted while driving and more used to taking risks.

New drivers with ADHD are even more likely to drive dangerously. Teen drivers with ADHD have a 62 percent higher risk for car crashes the first month after getting their license, compared to those without ADHD. In the first four years of driving, they have a 37 percent higher risk of being in a car accident, regardless of their age. Experts recommend that parents and adults spend extra time supervising young drivers with ADHD as they learn to drive and to limit the number of passengers in the car to limit distractions.

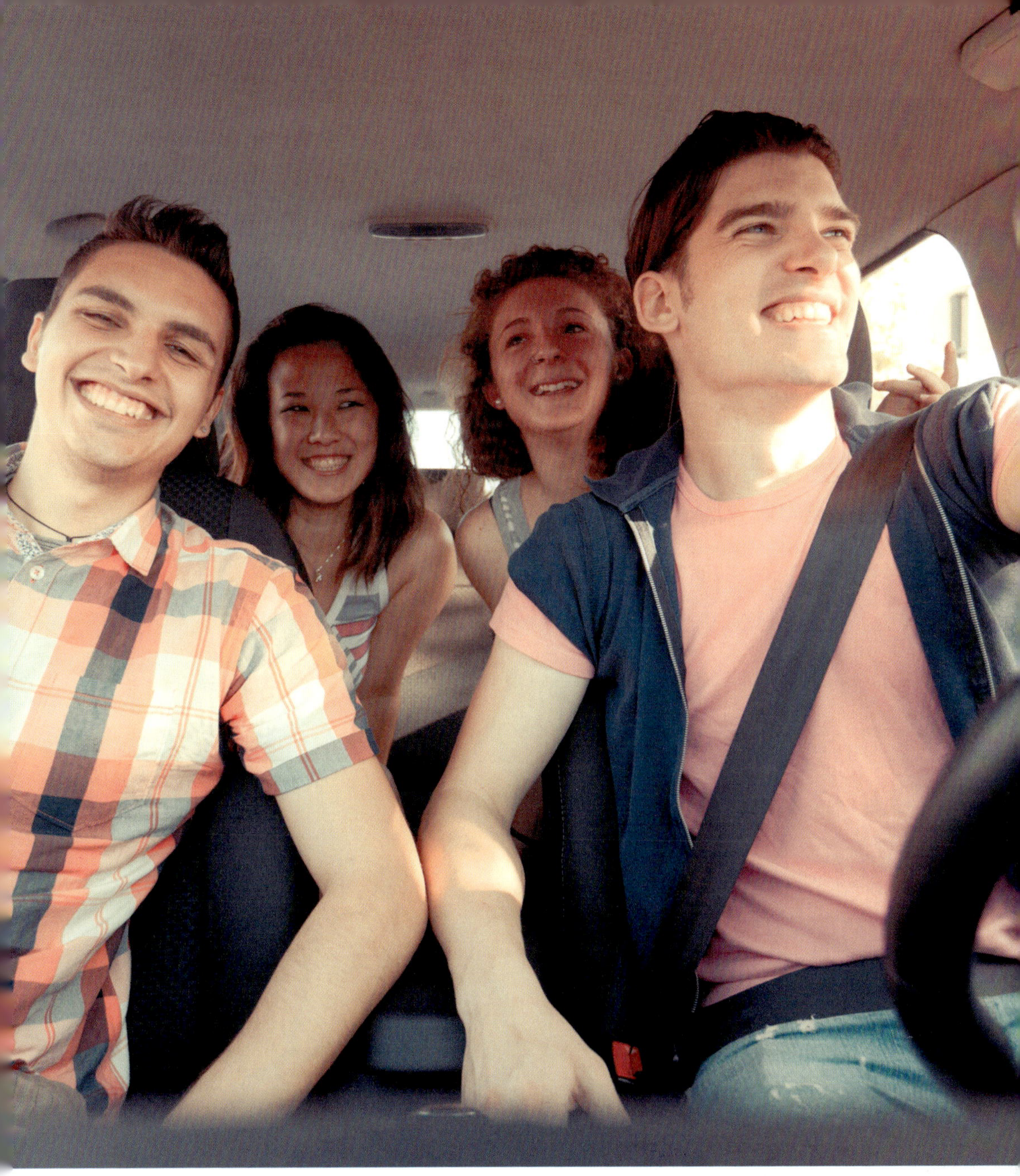

Distraction can create additional risk for teen drivers with ADHD.
They should be aware of this potential risk and take steps to lessen it.

have serious problems with peer relationships. Many children
with ADHD have trouble making and keeping friends due to
the inattention and impulsivity that is characteristic of ADHD.

They may interrupt or not listen to friends, fail to follow directions and play by the rules, and struggle to pick up on important social clues. Many children and adolescents with ADHD are easily frustrated and can have difficulty controlling their emotions. All of this can lead to conflicts with peers. The lack of success in the social domain in childhood can extend to the teen years, when the importance of friendships often increases. According to studies, adolescents and teens with ADHD have fewer friends and are more likely to be ignored or rejected by their peers, compared to those without the disorder. They also are more likely to be bullied or to bully others.

Other relationships suffer, too. According to Passmore, "Unfortunately, peer relationships are not the only relationships that experience a great deal of pressure. For children and adolescents with ADHD, family conflict is fairly common, and the more severe the symptoms, the more strained the relationships."[19] In one survey of 131 children with ADHD and their families, parents reported that their child's problems caused them emotional worry and limited the time they had to meet their own needs. Some of the conflict

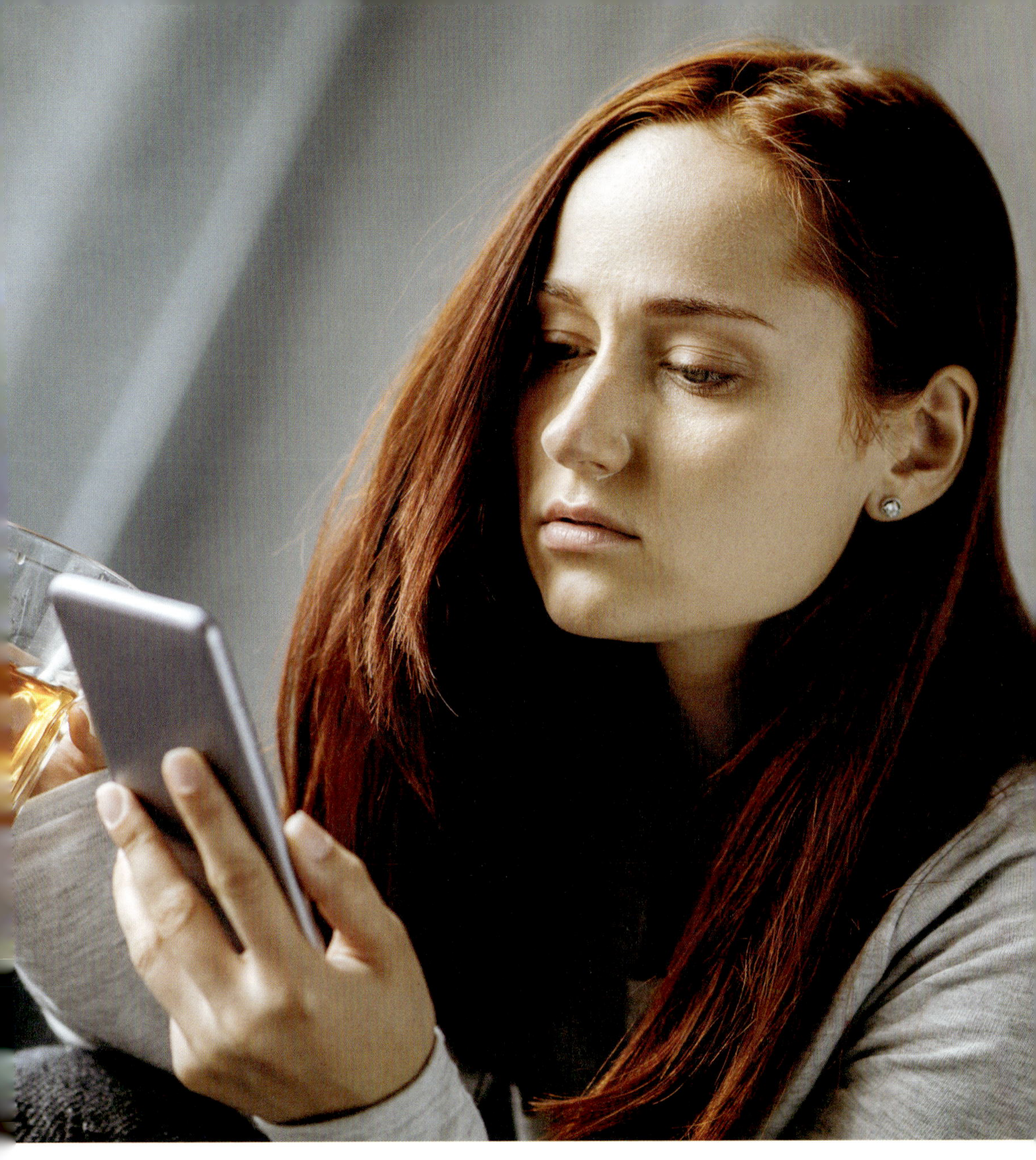

Teens with ADHD are at an elevated risk to partake in unsafe behaviors. On average, individuals with ADHD begin using alcohol at an earlier age and are more likely to suffer from alcohol dependence later on in their lives.

may be due to the adolescent's low tolerance for frustration

and difficulty regulating emotions. Also, teens and others with

ADHD can experience difficulties with household routines

and responsibilities, such as waking up on time, completing chores, and keeping their bedroom and belongings organized. This can lead to family conflicts. Some teens with ADHD also have oppositional defiant disorder or conduct disorder. These disorders are characterized by frequent conflict with parents or other authority figures, and that can lead to greater strains in family life.

RISKY BEHAVIORS

The teen years are a time of experimentation and pushing of boundaries as teens separate from parents to gain independence and more control over decision making. Engaging in risky behaviors is common for many teens and young adults, but the risks are higher for teens with ADHD. Research shows that teens with ADHD, as a group, start using alcohol, nicotine products, and illegal drugs earlier than teens without ADHD. This leads to higher rates of smoking, substance abuse, and alcohol-related problems in adults with ADHD. In addition, studies indicate that teens with ADHD tend to become sexually active earlier than those without the disorder, are more likely to have unsafe sex, and have higher rates of sexually transmitted diseases.

Teens with ADHD may be more apt to engage in risky behaviors for a number of reasons. Impaired impulsivity control

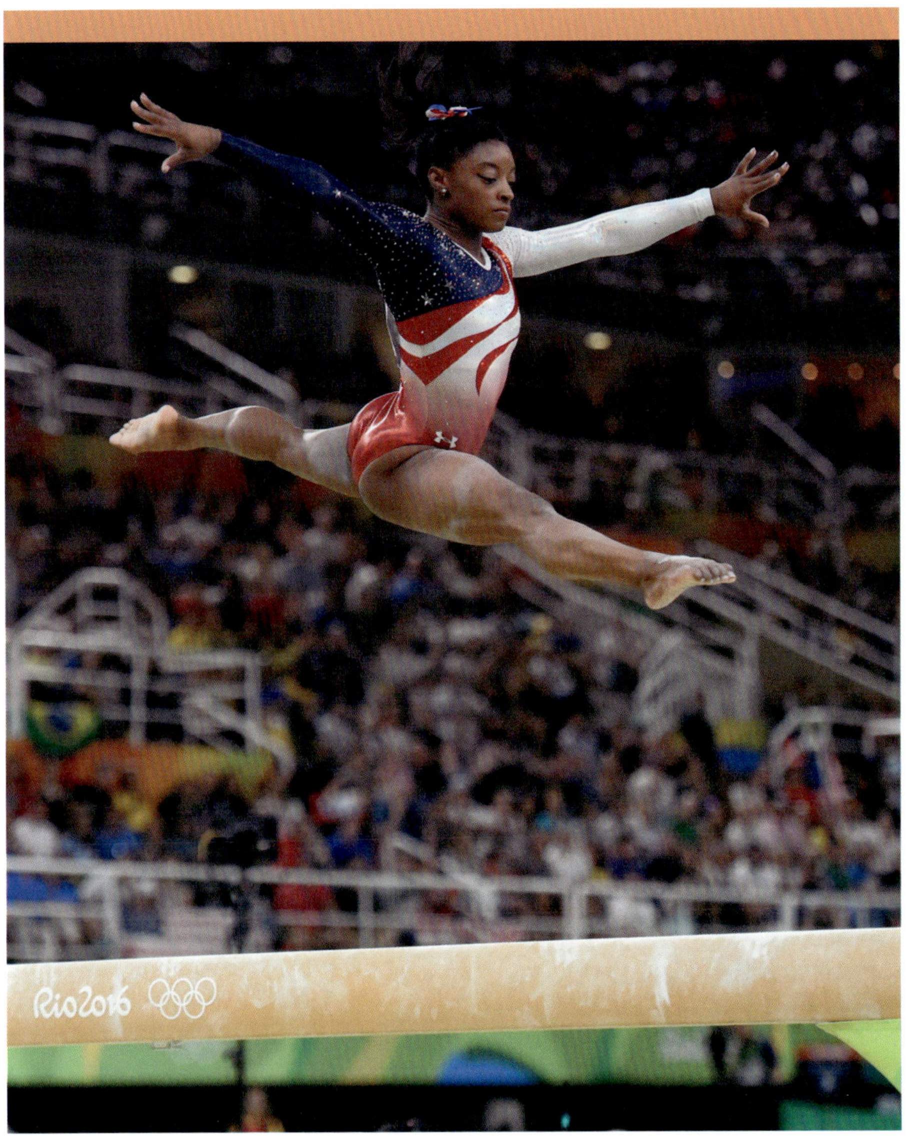

Olympic gymnast Simone Biles is one of many high-profile people who have ADHD. She has spoken out about knocking down the stigma associated with the disorder.

means that they are more likely to do something without thinking through the consequences. Also, teens who struggle with friendships and feelings of belonging may be more susceptible to peer pressure. Others may turn to alcohol and other substances to self-medicate the negative feelings associated with ADHD, such as low self-esteem.

BENEFITS

There certainly are risks associated with ADHD as teens move through high school and into adulthood. Many teens, however, can turn some of their ADHD traits to their advantage. ADHD can result in high levels of energy, which can be channeled toward success in many arenas, such as school, hobbies, jobs, and sports. Due to the different ways their brains process information, as well as the experience of living with the disorder, people with ADHD have a unique perspective on life. This can encourage creative and innovative approaches to tasks. Some people with ADHD find that they can become very focused when working on some tasks. Thomas E. Brown says, "Everyone I've ever evaluated for ADHD has some domains of activity where they can pay attention without difficulty."[20] Chesner notes the benefit of this hyperfocus: "A lot of special brains become really successful because they become almost obsessed with learning or achieving something."[21] Some successful adults who have been diagnosed with ADHD include musician Adam Levine, comedian Whoopi Goldberg, and gymnast Simone Biles. After winning four gold medals in the 2016 Olympics, Biles tweeted: "Having ADHD, and taking medicine for it is nothing to

be ashamed of."[22] Many teens
with ADHD become successful
and productive adults. Early
and accurate diagnosis, along
with a careful treatment and
management plan, can help
make this happen.

"Having ADHD, and taking
medicine for it is nothing to be
ashamed of."[22]

—Simone Biles,
Olympic gymnast

CHAPTER FOUR

How Is ADHD Treated and Managed?

There is no cure for ADHD. For the negative effects, there are a variety of treatment and management options available, including medication, behavior therapy, and alternative treatments. Individuals will respond to different treatment plans depending on their diagnosis and other factors. For example, children, whose brains are still developing, will require different treatments than adults. According to the CDC, "In most cases, ADHD is best treated with a combination of behavior therapy and medication."[23] A study of nearly 600 children with ADHD by the National Institutes of Health (NIH) also concluded that in many areas of functioning, including academic performance, parent-child relations, and social skills, "combination treatment was consistently superior to routine community care, whereas medication alone or behavior treatment alone were not."[24] Medication manages the brain-based functions and symptoms.

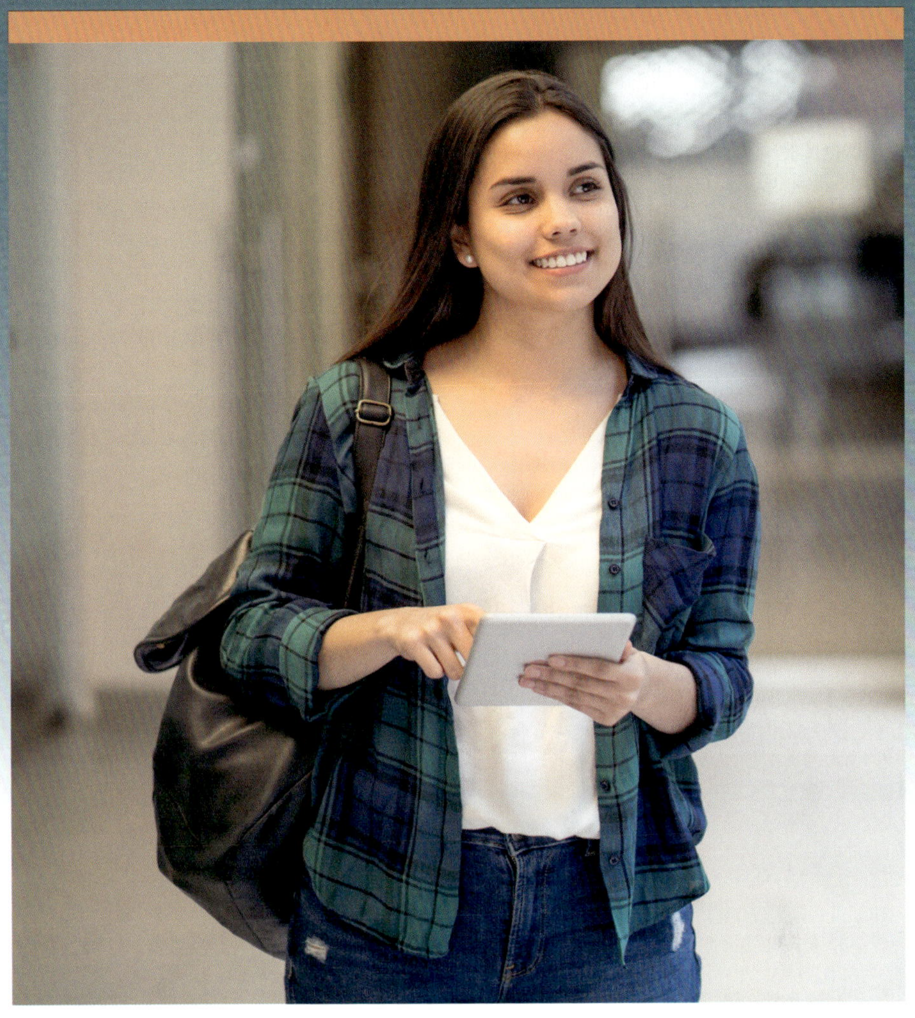

ADHD cannot be cured, but there are treatments and methods that make ADHD more manageable. People with ADHD are able to live healthy and successful lives.

Behavior therapy helps individuals with ADHD manage their daily thoughts and behaviors and develop positive coping strategies. Mental health professionals are trained to guide patients in the development of individualized treatment plans that work best for them.

The goal of all treatment and management plans is to control symptoms and allow people to live well. Successful treatment plans help teens improve functioning in school and work, benefit peer and family relationships, and decrease the risk of accidents and substance abuse.

MEDICATION

Medication is the most effective treatment for ADHD symptoms because it helps the brain function better. Medication helps people with ADHD feel more in control of how they act and think, and it allows them to focus and pay attention better. Common medications prescribed for ADHD symptoms include stimulants and some types of hypertension and antidepressant medications. Doctors prescribe medications for ADHD as they would any other medical condition. "Prescribing medication for an ADHD child is no different from prescribing insulin for a diabetic," says psychiatrist Dr. Ronald Kamm.[25]

Stimulants are the most common medications used to treat ADHD because studies have shown them to be the most effective for most patients. For many people, stimulants reduce hyperactivity and impulsivity and improve their ability to focus, work, and learn. Simulants have been used for decades in children and adults and are known to be among the safest of all psychiatric drugs. In addition, there is no evidence that the use of prescribed stimulants leads to drug abuse or dependence. Two commonly used stimulant medications are methylphenidate, which goes by different brand names, including Ritalin, and a combination of levoamphetamine and dextroamphetamine, known commercially as Adderall.

It may seem odd to treat ADHD with stimulants. According to Stuart Passmore, "Stimulant medication increases the arousal level of the central nervous system, and for many people with a hyperactive child, this seems to be an absurd approach."[26] Experts know, however, that the central nervous system (CNS) of a person with ADHD is actually less active that it should be. The CNS is the combination of the entire brain and the spinal cord. Stimulants work by boosting two important neurotransmitters: dopamine and norepinephrine. These chemical messengers are found throughout the brain. Once the medication begins to work, the CNS returns to a normal level of functioning. As a result, ADHD symptoms decrease.

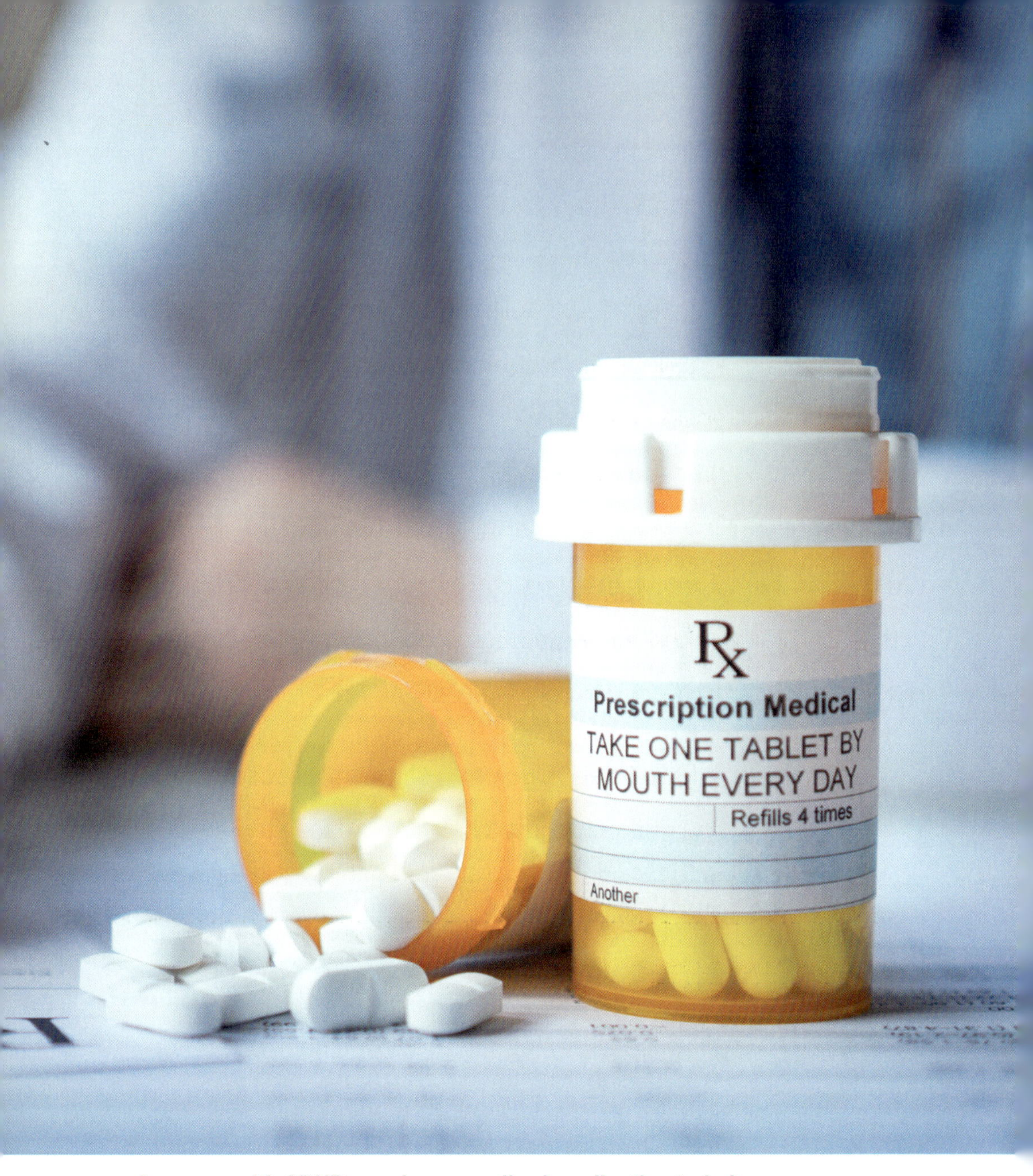

A person with ADHD may be prescribed medication to help manage symptoms. Because everyone responds to medication differently, it is important to have an individualized plan that is approved by a doctor.

About 10 to 20 percent of children with ADHD are not helped

by stimulants. Some people also experience negative effects

from the medication. Common side effects include insomnia

and feeling tired and sleepy in the middle of the day. Other side effects include high blood pressure and heart rate and personality changes. Stimulants also can suppress appetite, which might lead to weight loss and growth problems in children. If stimulants aren't a good fit for the patient, doctors might prescribe hypertension medications, which are generally used to treat high blood pressure, or antidepressants. Another challenge with medication is adherence, or the patient actually taking the medication as frequently as prescribed by the doctor. Side effects, stigma, and needing to take medication multiple times a day have been linked to lower adherence. Using medications that need to be taken less frequently has been linked to higher adherence.

NONMEDICAL TREATMENTS

A variety of nonmedical interventions have been shown to be effective in treating ADHD symptoms. Some of these treatments include behavior therapy, parental behavior training, and classroom interventions. Behavior therapy, also known as behavior modification, is designed to help adolescents and teens become responsible for their own behavior. They learn to recognize when they're acting inappropriately, and then they use skills and strategies they've learned to address the behavior. According to the CDC, "Behavior therapy is an effective treatment for attention-deficit/hyperactivity disorder (ADHD) that can improve a child's behavior, self-control, and self-esteem."[27] Behavior therapy is not a quick fix. It takes time and commitment and often involves participation by family members, teachers, and mental health professionals. The payoff is improved functioning at school, at home, and in social situations. According to a survey of children diagnosed with ADHD in 2014, six out of ten had received some type of behavior treatment.

Behavior therapy addresses specific problem behaviors associated with ADHD, such as difficulty getting to school on time or forgetting homework. The individual and parents or other caregivers set up clear rules and routines to increase success and reward good behavior. Experts recommend working on one goal at a time to avoid frustration. For example, if school tardiness is the behavior to be modified, the person would avoid trying to tackle a long list of goals at once. That full list might include setting a certain bedtime, starting homework immediately after school, making the bed every morning, getting up at 7:00, and being dressed by 7:30 in the morning as goals. Instead, the person would choose the top priority—perhaps getting out of bed at a certain time—and focus on that goal. Families create

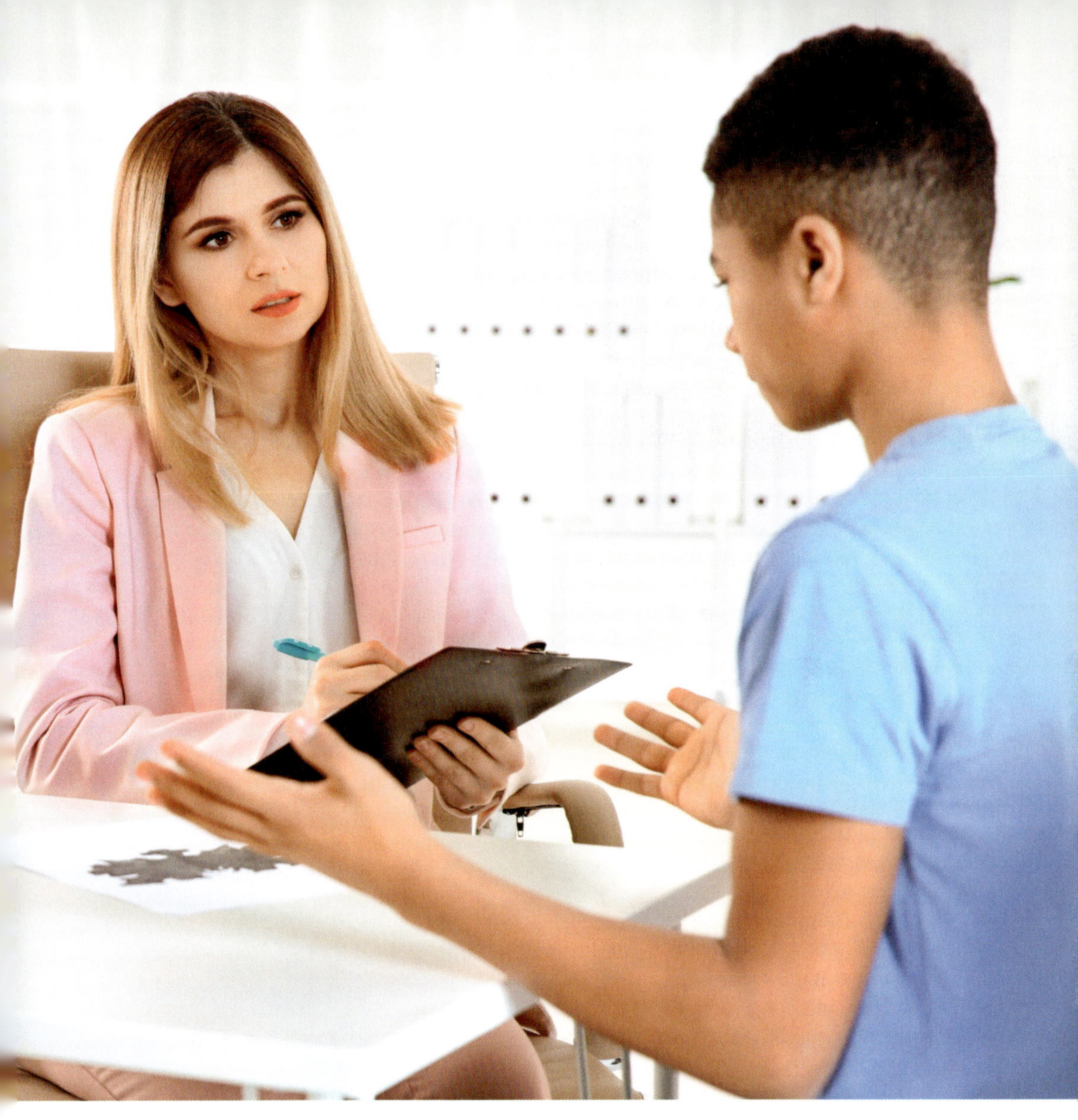

Behavior therapy can be especially helpful for people with ADHD. They will learn how to set goals and create strategies that will help them succeed.

routines that make the morning go more smoothly, and the teen is rewarded for getting up on time. Behavior therapy also helps people work through emotionally difficult situations and teaches strategies to control anger, cool down when frustrated, or think before speaking or acting.

For teens with more extreme emotional problems, cognitive behavioral therapy or dialectical behavior therapy can help. Both therapies focus on how thoughts, feelings, and behaviors influence one another. The therapies teach individuals how to accept their feelings and how to use coping strategies and positive thinking to change outcomes. These interventions combine behavioral therapy with mindfulness techniques or meditation, which focus on staying present in the moment and accepting thoughts and feelings without judgment.

Parenting does not cause ADHD. According to Passmore, "At one point in history when a child misbehaved in public or at school, the finger or blame was squarely pointed toward the parents, or more precisely at the child's

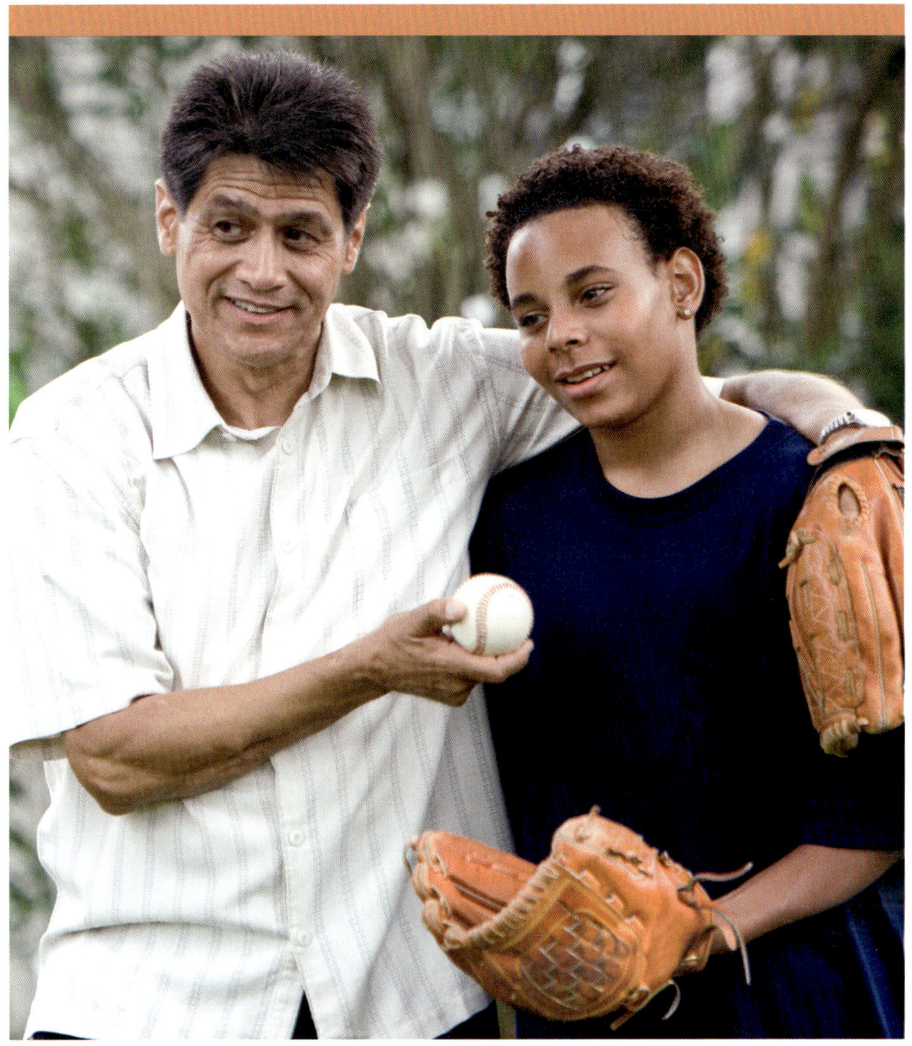

Parenting can make a big difference for kids with ADHD. Parents who understand what their kids are going through will be better able to support them.

mother."[28] The evidence about ADHD does not support this idea. Studies have shown, however, that children and teens with ADHD do benefit from particular parenting techniques, which parental behavior training can teach. Parental behavior training helps parents better understand ADHD, how it affects their child, and how best to help. It teaches parents how to structure the home and other situations to promote positive behavior and how to encourage and reward the desired behavior. They also learn techniques for ignoring or redirecting negative behaviors.

Classroom and academic interventions help adolescents and teens with ADHD by altering learning environments to make it easier to stay focused and complete work. Many of these interventions are simple, such as allowing the student to sit at the front of the class where it is easier to focus or providing a quiet place to complete homework or take a test. Teachers also may allow students with ADHD to take frequent breaks or to split larger assignments down into smaller, more manageable chunks. Students with an ADHD diagnosis may receive extended time to complete homework or tests. Also, they may be assigned a tutor or a peer to help with note taking in class and with homework.

Schools are required to provide accommodations because ADHD is recognized as a disability under the Americans with Disabilities Act. In 2014, nine out of ten children diagnosed with ADHD received school support. Fortunately for college-bound students, academic support doesn't end with high school. According to Elizabeth C. Hamblet, a learning specialist at Columbia University, "The encouraging truth is that all colleges— from community colleges through Ivy League schools—have to

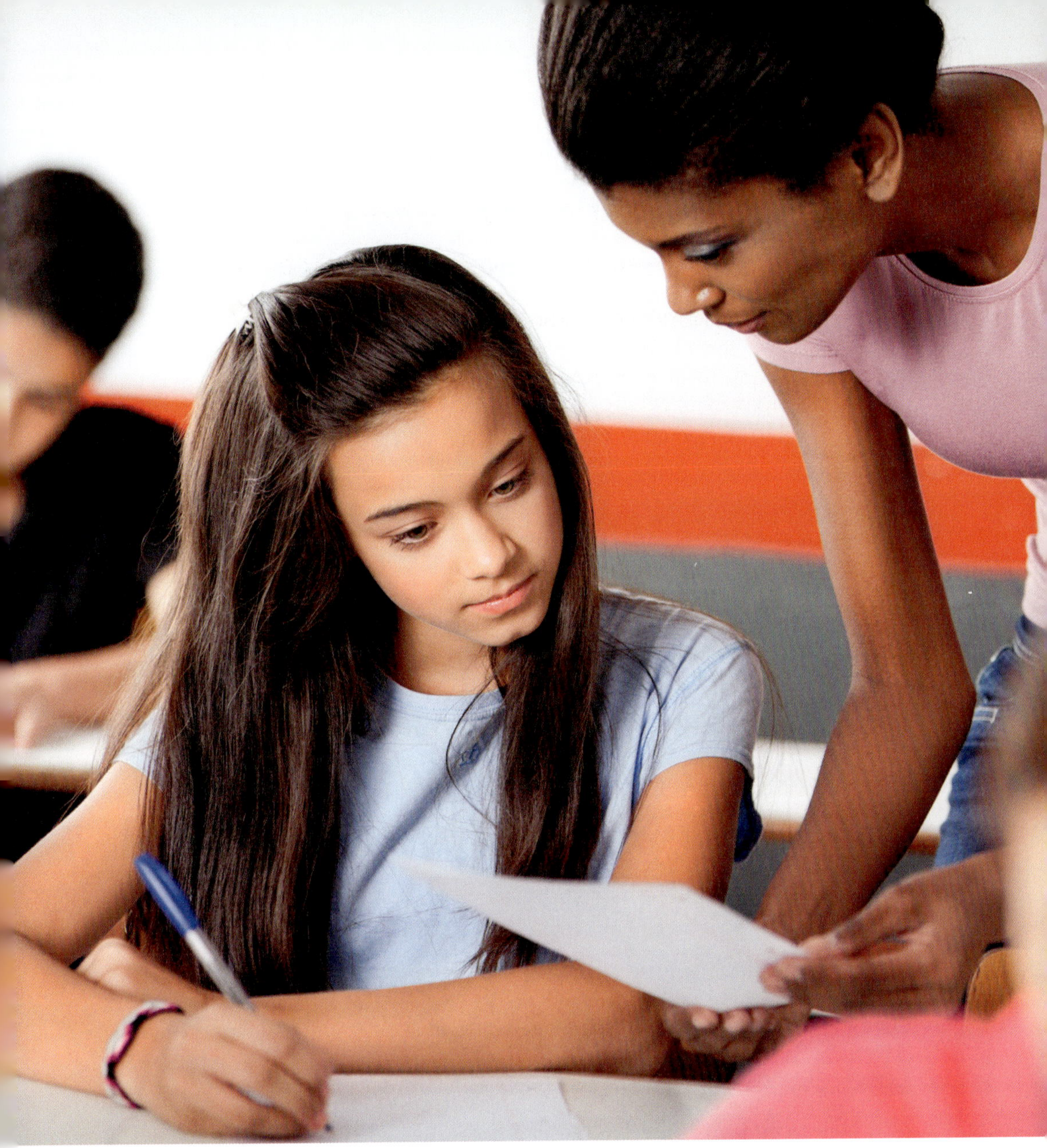

Teachers can take steps to help students who have ADHD. These interventions can help students remain focused and complete their assignments.

provide some accommodations for students with ADHD."[29] Still,

in some cases students do not request such accommodations,

and sometimes the accommodations for students with ADHD

are ineffective. Research continues on ways to make education more effective for those with ADHD.

MANAGING ADHD SYMPTOMS

"The encouraging truth is that all colleges—from community colleges through Ivy League schools—have to provide some accommodations for students with ADHD."[29]

—Elizabeth C. Hamblet, learning specialist at Columbia University

A combination of medical and nonmedical interventions is most effective in treating ADHD symptoms. In addition, adolescents and teens can employ a number of strategies to help manage their symptoms on a daily basis. These methods can help improve academic, social, and emotional functioning in everyday life. Because each person with ADHD is unique, some methods will be more effective than others for different people.

To improve functioning in all areas, particularly at home and school, experts highly recommend that teens with ADHD have good routines and predictable schedules. Posting a schedule in a visible place, such as the kitchen, will remind teens of important appointments, activities, and academic due dates. Schedules and routines add structure to the day, which can be helpful if inattention, memory, and impulsivity are an issue. Organization is another good management tool. Have a place for everything in the house and always put items away. This results

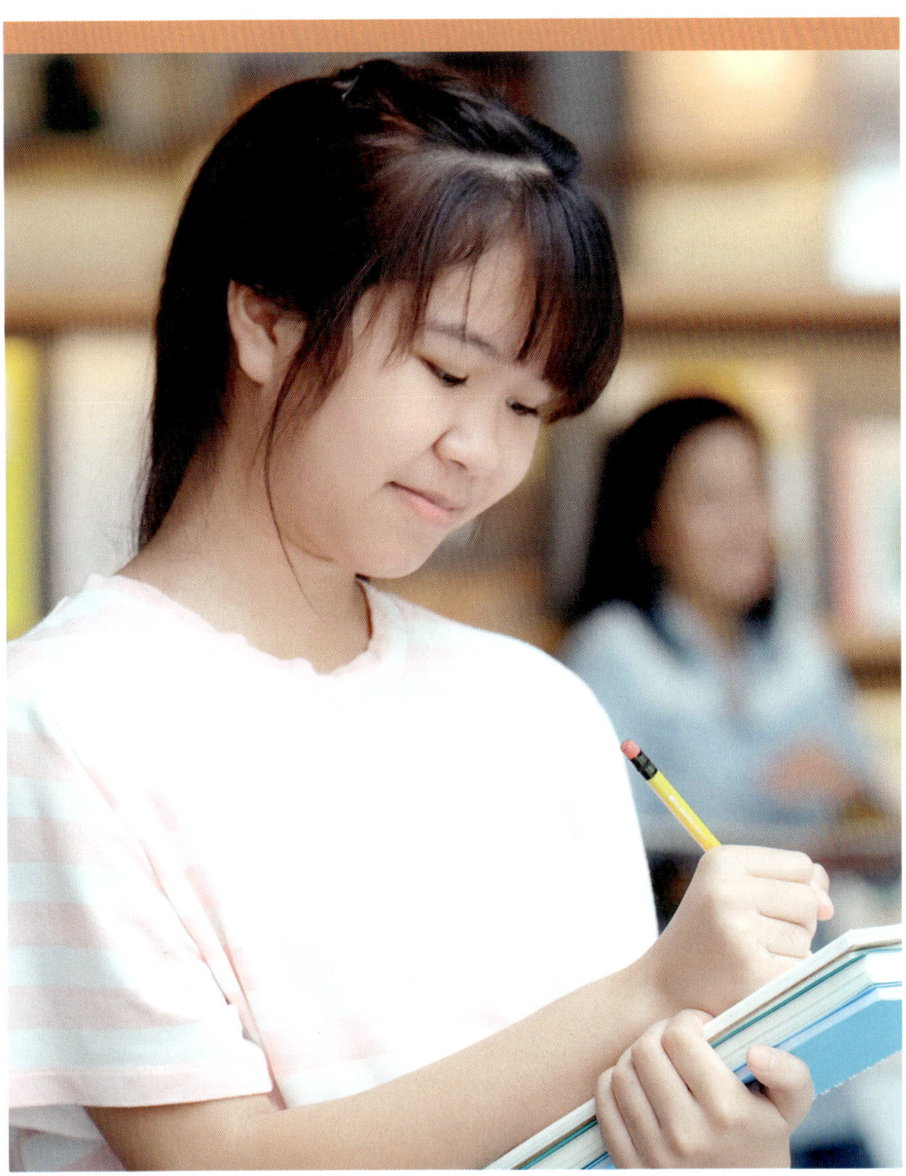

Having a set schedule or routine helps with organization. This structure helps someone with ADHD manage her life and prioritize different tasks.

in fewer important things lost, such as homework and car keys. It also reduces the frustration that results from searching for lost items, especially when it's time to leave the house for school or an activity. Experts recommend that teens use homework and notebook organizers for schoolwork. Students are encouraged to write down tests, assignments, and required books and materials in a daily schedule and to get in the habit of checking the schedule before leaving home in the morning and before leaving school in the afternoon. Many other strategies can help adolescents and teens self-manage their symptoms. These include eating healthful foods and not skipping meals, exercising daily to improve health and relieve stress, and getting plenty of sleep at night. It can also be helpful to build in relaxation time to relieve feelings of frustration and stress. And, finally, experts recommend that teens with ADHD stay away from alcohol and drugs, which can make impulsivity symptoms worse.

If a teen is struggling with friendships and other peer relationships, he or she should talk with a parent or other trusted adult. Therapists also can help teach positive social skills. Structured social activities, such as extracurricular activities, sports, and clubs, can offer opportunities for positive peer interactions.

Kids and teens with ADHD sometimes have trouble staying positive and may struggle with low self-esteem. They may focus on negative feelings, such as shame, failure, and chronic stress. Studies have found, however, that positive thinking can lead to better mental health. According to John F. Taylor, "Scientists have proven it in experiments. People who think positively are more likely to feel good about themselves."[30] To regulate strong negative emotions, some experts recommend a strengths-based approach. This means thinking about what is right, not what is wrong. Adolescents and teens are encouraged to focus on their strengths and the positive traits that ADHD can bring, such as creativity, energy, and drive. Group therapy and peer support groups can help teens process and cope with negative feelings.

ADHD can be a difficult disorder for anyone diagnosed, and it can be particularly challenging for teens. The good news is that recognition of ADHD as a medical condition that has brain-based causes is growing. Along with a better understanding of the disorder comes better diagnosis and more targeted treatments for the negative symptoms. Many teens learn to not just live but thrive with ADHD.

Source Notes

Introduction: Unable to Focus

1. "ADHD Data and Statistics," *Centers for Disease Control and Prevention*, October 15, 2019. www.cdc.gov.

2. "Evidence-Based Therapies," *Society of Clinical Child & Adolescent Psychology*, April 24, 2018. https://effectivechildtherapy.org.

Chapter 1: What Is ADHD?

3. Quoted in "Symptoms and Diagnosis of ADHD," *Centers for Disease Control and Prevention*, November 1, 2019. www.cdc.gov.

4. John F. Taylor, *The Survival Guide for Kids with ADD or ADHD*. Minneapolis, MN: Free Spirit Publishing, 2006. p. 15.

5. "Attention-Deficit/Hyperactivity Disorder (ADHD) in Children: Overview," *Mayo Clinic,* n.d. www.mayoclinic.org.

6. "What Is Attention-Deficit/Hyperactivity Disorder?," *Centers for Disease Control and Prevention*, n.d. www.cdc.gov.

Chapter 2: What Causes ADHD and How Is It Diagnosed?

7. "The Science of ADHD," *Children and Adults with Attention-Deficit/Hyperactivity Disorder*, 2020. www.chadd.org.

8. Larry Silver, "The Neuroscience of the ADHD Brain," *ADDitude*, August 12, 2019. www.additudemag.com.

9. Jonathan Chesner, *ADHD in HD: Brains Gone Wild*. Minneapolis, MN: Free Spirit Publishing, 2012. p. 6.

10. Thomas E. Brown, "The Adult ADHD Mind: Executive Function Connections," *Additude*, April 1, 2006. https://arc.duke.edu.

11. Chesner, *ADHD in HD: Brains Gone Wild*, p. 6.

12. Chesner, *ADHD in HD: Brains Gone Wild*, p. 6.

Chapter 3: What Is It like to Live With ADHD?

13. "About ADHD—Overview," *Children and Adults with Attention-Deficit/Hyperactivity Disorder*, 2020. www.chadd.org.

14. Stan Kutcher, "ADHD: Attention Deficit Hyperactivity Disorder," *TeenMentalHealth Speaks Magazine*, September 15, 2019. p. 6.

15. Kutcher, "ADHD: Attention Deficit Hyperactivity Disorder," p. 6.

16. Stuart Passmore, *The ADHD Handbook*. Wollombi, Australia: Exisle Publishing, 2014. p. 189.

17. Kutcher, "ADHD: Attention Deficit Hyperactivity Disorder," p. 17.

18. Chesner, *ADHD in HD: Brains Gone Wild*, p. 31.

19. Passmore, *The ADHD Handbook*, p. 6.

20. Brown, "The Adult ADHD Mind: Executive Function Connections."

21. Chesner, *ADHD in HD: Brains Gone Wild*, p. 49.

22. Maxwell Strachan, "Simone Biles Proudly Opens Up About Having ADHD," *HuffPost*, September 16, 2016. www.huffpost.com.

Chapter 4: How Is ADHD Treated and Managed?

23. "What Is Attention-Deficit/Hyperactivity Disorder?"

24. "The Multimodal Treatment of Attention Deficit Hyperactivity Disorder Study," *National Institute of Mental Health*, November 2009. nimh.nih.gov.

25. Quoted in Aimee Crawford, "Bravo, Simone Biles, for Taking a Stand Against ADHD Stigma," *ESPN*, September 21, 2016. www.espn.com.

26. Passmore, *The ADHD Handbook*, p. 106.

27. "Parent Training," *Centers for Disease Control and Prevention*, September 30, 2019. www.cdc.gov.

28. Passmore, *The ADHD Handbook*, p. 142.

29. Elizabeth C. Hamblet, "What Students with ADHD and Their Parents Should Know About College," *Attention Magazine*, December 2013. www.chadd.org.

30. Taylor, *The Survival Guide for Kids with ADD or ADHD*, p. 20.

Books

Carla Mooney, *Teens and ADHD*. San Diego, CA: ReferencePoint Press, 2017.

John Perritano, *ADHD and Other Behavior Disorders*. Broomall, PA: Mason Crest, 2018.

Whitney Sanderson, *Living with ADHD*. San Diego, CA: ReferencePoint Press, 2018.

Internet Sources

Thomas E. Brown, "The Adult ADHD Mind: Executive Function Connections," *ADDitude*, April 1, 2006. https://arc.duke.edu.

"International Consensus Statement on ADHD," *Clinical Child and Family Psychology Review*, Vol. 5, No. 2, June 2002. www.russellbarkley.org.

Rachel Nall, "The Benefits of ADHD," *Healthline*, January 25, 2016. www.healthline.com.

Larry Silver, "The Neuroscience of the ADHD Brain," *ADDitude*, August 12, 2019. www.additudemag.com.

Websites

Attention Deficit Disorder Association (ADDA)
www.add.org

The website of the ADDA provides information, resources, and networking opportunities for adults with ADHD.

Centers for Disease Control and Prevention (CDC)
www.cdc.gov/ncbddd/adhd/index.html

The CDC's website on ADHD provides information on the facts, symptoms, diagnosis, and treatment of ADHD. It also reports recent research and data, statistics on the disorder, and scientific articles and recommendations for diagnosis and treatment.

Children and Adults with Attention-Deficit/ Hyperactivity Disorder (CHADD)
www.chadd.org

This website contains evidence-based information on ADHD as well as advocacy and resources for support for children and adults with ADHD.

Teen Mental Health
https://teenmentalhealth.org

This website contains information and resources on a number of mental health issues for teens, their families, and educators, including ADHD. The site focuses on the most recent evidence-based medicine and research.

Index

Index Continued

Image Credits

Cover: © Cagkan Sayin/Shutterstock Images

5: © Antonio_Diaz/iStockphoto

6: © Syda Productions/Shutterstock Images

9: © Syda Productions/Shutterstock Images

11: © baona/iStockphoto

15: © KatarzynaBialasiewicz/iStockphoto

16: © Monkey Business Images/Shutterstock Images

19: © Rawpixel/iStockphoto

21: © Sebastian Kaulitzki/Shutterstock Images

23: © Billion Photos/Shutterstock Images

25: © Wavebreakmedia/iStockphoto

27: © Phovoir/Shutterstock Images

32: © PeopleImages/iStockphoto

35: © Monkey Business Images/Shutterstock Images

36: © SDI Productions/iStockphoto

39: © LightFieldStudios/iStockphoto

42: © fizkes/Shutterstock Images

44: © Syda Productions/Shutterstock Images

47: © William Perugini/Shutterstock Images

49: © yacobchuk/iStockphoto

51: © A.RICARDO/Shutterstock Images

55: © Hispanolistic/iStockphoto

58: © erdikocak/iStockphoto

61: © New Africa/Shutterstock Images

63: © Golden Pixels LLC/Shutterstock Images

65: © Tyler Olson/Shutterstock Images

67: © mangpor2004/Shutterstock Images

Yvette LaPierre lives in North Dakota with her family and teaches writing at the University of North Dakota. She writes and edits books and articles for children and adults.